Ageless Beauty

The Ultimate Skincare & Makeup Book for Women & Teens of Color

Ageless Beauty

The Ultimate Skincare & Makeup Book for Women & Teens of Color

Alfred Fornay
and Yvonne Rose

Amber Books
Phoenix
New York   Los Angeles

Ageless Beauty
The Ultimate Skincare & Makeup Book
for Women and Teens of Color
by Alfred Fornay
and Yvonne Rose

Published by:
Amber Communications Group, Inc.
1334 East Chandler Boulevard, Suite 5-D67
Phoenix, AZ 85048
Phone: 602-743-7211
Email: amberbk@aol.com
www.amberbooks.com

Tony Rose, Publisher / Editorial Director
Yvonne Rose, Associate Publisher/Senior Editor
Yvonne Shackleford, Associate Editor
Mercedes Fleetwood, Beauty Column
The Printed Page, Cover Layout & Interior Design

ISBN#: 978-0-9790976-8-3

Library of Congress Cataloging-in-Publication Data

Fornay, Alfred.
  Ageless beauty : the skincare & makeup guide for women and teens of color / by Alfred Fornay with Yvonne Rose.
     p. cm.
  ISBN 978-0-9790976-8-3
1. Skin--Care and hygiene. 2. African American women--Health and hygiene. 3. Teenage girls--Health and hygiene. 4. African American teenagers--Health and hygiene. 5. Beauty, Personal. I. Rose, Yvonne. II. Title.
  RL87.F665 2011
  646.7'2608996073--dc22
                    2011013494

Dedication

This book is dedicated to all women of color, past, present and future, who strive for excellence in their work, family and personal grooming. You have taught us to respect and appreciate your *Ageless Beauty*.

Table of Contents

Beauty is Ageless, neither young nor old, but eternal!

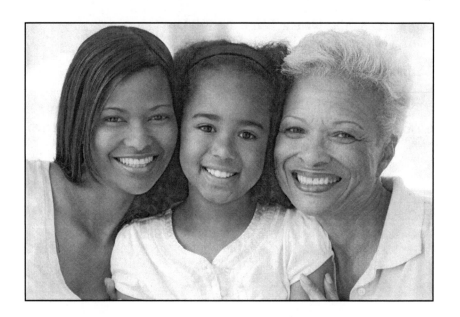

Introduction

Ageless Beauty is for women and teenagers whose skin tones come in a multitude of complexions. Reading Ageless Beauty will teach you how to understand your skin. You will learn how to take care of your skin so that it takes care of you and how to transform it from a blotchy bother to an ageless accessory. You will also learn secretly-traded techniques to nourishing your skin so that it not only turns your head when you see your reflection, but it also turns the heads of your admirers and friends every time you walk by!

Ageless Beauty reaffirms and defines beauty for women and teenagers of color on your own terms. The time-honored techniques found in this book will help you look fabulous and feel beautiful just in time for your weekend plans. It is about the health and beauty of your skin, its maintenance, its treatment, its make-up, and it is about the application of color to your skin and nails. Wise women say you should learn something new every day…why not gain a little knowledge with a heaping side of undiscovered inner and outer beauty? The timeless techniques found between these pages have been proven to work for all stages of life. Imagine using the same regiment to maintain your youthful, pre-teen glow from your sweet 16 to your first birthday with triple digits without skipping a beat?

Ageless Beauty is an easy-to-follow guide for ethnic women and teenagers just like you, whether you are a manager of a small service store, a student, or an executive of a multi-million dollar corporation. It is written for the stressed out office manager of a small business who is also a new wife and mother of three; it is written for the editor of a major magazine who is a part-time student in the evenings working on a master's degree; it is for the high school freshman who wants to start wearing make-up; it is for the domestic engineer whose jobs are innumerable and whose hours are unending; it is for the single mother who just earned her bachelor's degree, was recently laid off, and is on a hunt to find employment to provide for her family. This book is easy reading with simple concepts that can be realistically added to your daily routine without taking more than a few extra moments of your already precious time.

Ageless Beauty is a guide about the beauty of your heritage that speaks to all women and teenagers of color, from every background. While you may recognize that your ancestral roots are in Africa, you have most likely turned to some aspect of our modern times to create a culture of fashion and style that is uniquely yours. Your face reveals a melting pot of your heritage that was shaped centuries ago by your Native American, Asian, Latin, and African ancestors. Your profile includes the gentle blending of dark hues and fair hues with bold and wonderful features, brown skin freckled from the sun, brown and hazel eyes peeking through ebony lashes. You have exciting potential that eagerly waits to be discovered and nurtured so that you become a more attractive, more interesting, more appealing you.

YOU are awesome! YOU are wonderful! YOU were born beautiful! YOU are an *Ageless Beauty!* Have fun learning how to bring out the attractive, appealing person you've dreamed about being. You'll learn everything you want to know about great skin, gorgeous makeup, chic hairstyles, and more.

o   YOU will learn how to evaluate the quality of the product lines that are being offered to you through department stores, chain stores, pharmacies and direct marketing companies

o   YOU will discover how to choose what works best for you, how to address your personal skin care needs and feel secure in your selection of products o   YOU will be able to determine your skin type and understand what colors are appropriate for your skin tone

o   YOU will know what regular skin care regimen to follow and, whenever necessary, what corrective beauty products to buy

Ageless Beauty is for all women and teens of multiple ethnicities who want to look great and take better care of their skin. Whether your skin color is chocolate, ivory, mocha, caramel or bronze, you should feel fabulous about yourself, look gorgeous every day, be as healthy as possible, and your beauty should be appreciated by yourself and other members of our wonderful global community. Ageless beauty is about YOU and for YOU!

—Yvonne Rose and Yvonne Shackleford

Chapter 1

How Your Skin Protects You

Your facial skin can be your best friend. It is your confidante. It is your protector. It takes all types of abuse, and yet it is quick and ready to forgive.

Your skin is a multifaceted creation that can't be duplicated by human beings. It keeps out the harsh external environment—that is, germs and bacteria—while it protects your vital organs. It helps maintain your body temperature by preventing heat from escaping too rapidly, which would lead to harm or even death.

Your skin is versatile and sensitive. It reacts to stress, pain, illness, pleasure, happiness, and to light and dark, hot and cold. It stretches and shrinks, wrinkles and unwrinkles. It needs minimal but regular, consistent, and thorough attention if you want it to show you at your very best. But for all your skin's strength and versatility, today it is under siege. It is bombarded by more natural and unnatural stresses than were ever intended.

Geography and the Seasons

Where you live has a direct effect on your skin, particularly on your face, for it is almost always exposed to the elements. Your face has an upper, or outer, layer of skin called the epidermis. This layer is what you touch and see when you look in the mirror. Actually, it is a series of layers, each somewhat different from the one above it but all with enough in common that together they make up the epidermis. Another name for this layer, owing to the shape of the cells making up the layers, is the "horny" layer (stratum corneum).

Although everyone has this outer skin layer, the thickness of the covering differs from person to person. African Americans have more layers to their epidermis than do European Americans. But for all ethnicities, the number of layers varies. Now you can understand why your face, to some degree, reacts differently to the forces assaulting it than do the faces of other women you know.

The outermost portion of the epidermis consists of dead cells. That is why sometimes, after washing your face and drying it with a towel, you may notice flaking skin on your forehead. Your face casts off this outermost layer of skin in pieces. As the outer layer is dispelled, an under layer takes its place. This is a constantly renewing process. Each outermost layer falls away when it has absorbed all the stress it can manage, and then the under layer takes its place.

While this surface action is taking place, the under layer is protected, waiting to supply your face with a new fighting army of cells. Beneath the epidermis is the germinating layer, but before discussing this lower layer, let's see what geography and climate can do to the outer layer of your skin.

If you live in a year-round warm region like California, then your skin will be affected differently than if you live on the East Coast, in a climate that has four varying seasons. Obviously, there is a difference in the amount of the sun and ultraviolet rays that will attack your skin, based on where your home is. But this is only the beginning.

If you live in a very sunny climate, then generally the office buildings are air conditioned year-round. The same is true when you fly in a pressurized aircraft. Whether it's in the sky or on the ground, air-conditioning draws humidity from the air and moisture from the skin. So, by the time you go from your dry office into a sun-drenched day, to bombard your skin with ultraviolet rays and further draw off moisture, your skin has really taken a beating. The skin is left dry, peeling, and if the exposure was too intense, with its under layers damaged.

The effect of just these two factors—sun and air-conditioning—is significant and potentially serious. This is the damage that sunburns do: you peel or you're left with leathery-looking skin. Worse, this constant negative stress breaks down the face's connective tissue, resulting in wrinkles and "aging." With steady damage, those wrinkles and lines around the eyes and mouth begin getting deeper and more prominent.

If you live in a seasonal climate, you might feel safer—and to some degree, that is true. But in the East, often there are major industrial complexes nearby that spew pollutants into the air. And wherever you live or work, your skin is exposed to automobile emissions and wind. Wind alone can strike at your skin and cause damage, but when that wind carries pollutants, the problem is intensified. The pollutants that cause acid rain destroy forests and crops, so you can imagine the struggle your outer skin layer has to protect your body.

Central heating, as well as air-conditioning, dries out the skin. This instrument of comfort adds stress to your face and brings on a premature aging process. To some degree, the effects of the seasons—even geography —may not be as dangerous to your face as is the modern technology we've created to make our lives more comfortable.

Other natural assaults come from germs, bacteria, and environmental impurities. These elements also must be prevented from getting below the skin's surface. So no matter where you live, your face contends with major stresses. More often than not, the outer layer stands up to these assaults—but at a cost: dryness, wrinkles and lines, and skin disorders. Your skin can't fight the "good fight" alone; it needs your help.

Misinformation

Perhaps even more disturbing than the elements our skin is exposed to is the degree to which people are misinformed. Dark-skinned women and men have often been led to believe that their skin is built for the sun. Their African background is used as the factor to make this belief seem true. In fact, it is not true.

If you take a careful look at "blacks" living in the desert, or in comparably dry, hot regions like the Sudan, you will note that their bodies almost always are totally covered and very little of their skin is exposed to the sun. In contrast, people living in hot, humid areas are less apt to wear clothes, and rightfully so. Generally, the hot, humid areas have little if any direct pollutants, and the humidity in the air reduces the degree to which skin moisture evaporates. People who live in very humid climates don't peel; people with darker skin tones often have fewer wrinkles and they have faces that belie their age. The outer layer of their skin is moist and pliable, rather than dry and lined.

I've talked with women from Gabon and the Central African Republic, and they complain about how dry their skin becomes when they visit America. Their complaints have validity, since the humidity here is relatively low. A change in climate like this is often noticed within a few days or less. So remember—whatever your color, protect your skin or you will pay for the neglect.

Dark skin has special qualities. It has more epidermal layers than light skin. To some degree, this means greater protection from the sun and because of those additional layers, black skin often appears and feels smoother. Dark skin has more melanin (the dark pigment in the epidermis), which reflects more of the sun's rays, giving greater protection and reducing the drying process. But for all these positive qualities, dark skin needs as much care as any other if it is to maintain its health and good looks.

Devices of Protection

As previously stated, there are two upper layers to the skin: the epidermis and the germination layer, which together make up the skin's essential defense system. The outer layer has two essential ingredients helping it to do its job and maintain its "looks": water and sebaceous oils. These two elements—no matter how often you may have heard that oil and water don't mix—work together beautifully to support and protect the skin.

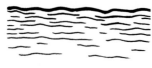

The upper layer of epithelial tissue, the under layer of germinating tissue, and the dermis, with regular blood cells.

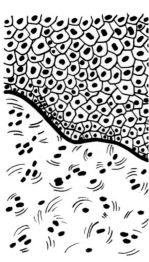

The epidermis needs water to keep it pliable, plump, and elastic. You need to drink plenty of water to maintain healthy skin. The sebaceous glands produce oils that travel upward and cover the surface of the skin. The oils act as a defensive shield and a reflector, holding the skin's surface moisture in and also keeping the skin soft, pliable, and unbroken. However, once moisture is drawn from the outer layer, the oils cannot help restore the skin's youthful quality. Only water will do the job. If you soak a piece of dry skin in oil, for example, it will not soften. It will not soften even if you use sebaceous oil. The oil is not the softener, water is. Remember this principle when we focus on products for your skin-care regimen.

The Germinating Layer

Beneath the epidermis is the germinating layer. Actually, this is the deepest layer of the epidermis, resting on the corium, which is also called the derma, or true skin. But the germinating layer is so different from the rest of the epidermis, and should be nurtured so differently, that I present it as though it were a distinct layer. It consists of a single row of columnar cells, in which young cells develop and move upward to the surface.

The top cells making up the germinating layer move upward while others remain, protecting the corium beneath. The germinating layer does not maintain itself on water or oils, but is nourished by the blood circulated to the skin. This layer of cells is nourished as are cells in the rest of your body, through proper nutrients. This is why what you eat and don't eat, what you take into your system and what you don't take into it, will show in your face. What gets into your circulatory system will be seen, one way or another. Drinking alcohol will show, smoking will show, drugs will show, birth-control pills will show. A healthful or poor diet will show. Your skin is an indicator of your state of health. Moreover, your state of health will either help or prevent your skin from doing its job.

The pH Defense

Those sebaceous glands have another defensive purpose besides holding in the skin's moisture. They maintain what is called an acid mantle across the skin's surface. Healthy skin is slightly acidic. It is believed that skin with a tendency toward alkalinity (the opposite of acidity) is more likely to become infected and have skin disorders. The pH factor of healthy skin (a tendency towards acidity) works as a defense, warding off infection and disorders that affect the skin's ability to both do its job and save the body from having to fight beneath the surface as well. So when you see products proclaiming to return the skin's pH factor, don't automatically accept or reject them, but know that the pH measure is important.

I have deliberately not discussed the skin's corium, or derma, since commercial products cannot affect it. Your genes, diet, and cosmetic surgery are its primary influences. So you can readily understand that the epidermis and germination layers with the sebaceous glands are the skin's primary, effective defense against the environment, both human—and nature-made. The "fall off" defensive process of the outermost layer of the epidermis serves two vital functions: (1) the older and drier cells are removed, and as the layer of the cells falls off, (2) the environmental impurities, bacteria, and pollutants on or in them are removed.

This self-renewing process is ongoing, with little visible evidence when your skin is young and healthy. However, when your skin is neither young nor healthy, then the process works less effectively, with the noticeable results of lines, wrinkles, cracks, and peeling. But with help and knowledge, you can retard the aging process and keep your skin healthy and youthful-looking.

Water—A Key To Youthful-Looking Skin

Even though the outer layer of the skin receives a continuous supply of water from the inner layer, the amount provided is limited at any given time. Thus, the outer layer is often short of water when it may need it most. For example, if the skin's loss of water to the atmosphere exceeds its upward supply, then the skin is in danger of going dry. If you don't use a sunscreen or moisturizing guard, the extreme dry conditions in such areas as Arizona, New Mexico, and the desert in California can have a dangerous effect on your skin.

The Aging Process

If you look at the skin of an older person, particularly if it has been neglected or abused, you will find evidence of structural change. The dead, outer layer of the epidermis is thicker and therefore drier. In part, this is because the epidermis begins to produce a slightly different type of cell.

Furthermore, these cells stick together with greater adhesion and are not shed as readily. The outer layers of dead skin begin to build up thicker and thicker atop the lower, living layers. These outer layers have not only less water or moisture in them but also less capacity to hold water. Unless their moisture capacity is increased, the outer, now thicker layer becomes dry and wrinkled. This causes creepy lines to appear, with the ends of the cells curling up, leading to roughness.

During this aging process, the oil glands decrease in function, with the decline greater in women than in men. Also, the surface guard of oil, whose function is to hold moisture in the skin, does not work as well. Without its water retention, the skin loses its pliability and softness. Finally, the outer layer may hold up to the point where rough, red spots appear and discolorations show up on black skin.

Suntanning and the Aging Process

Tanning is a device the skin uses to protect its delicate inner layers. This increase in pigment, brought about through exposure to sunlight, by and large is temporary; the suntan disappears in time. However, during the aging process, there is a tendency for these pigments to increase, causing the skin to become darker and, in some instances, blotchy. These darker areas usually appear on the hands and face. Often they are called age spots or liver spots, and they are permanent. Actually, these are the result of suntanning combined with the aging process. People who stay out of the sun have fewer, if any, liver spots.

Lines, Wrinkles, and Spots

If you were able to take a look at the skin's lower layer—the dermis —you would notice elastic fibers. The dermis cannot regenerate itself as can the epidermis, or outer layer. Any damage done to the dermis results in degeneration and the formation of scar tissue. This means there is a structural change, no matter how slight. It is this under layer that is reasonable for the resiliency of your facial skin, whether smooth and unlined or rough and wrinkled. The dermas is composed of layers of living tissue, and this tissue is permeated with elastic fibers—reinforcement rods that help keep the skin taut. If damage is done to these rods, sagging and wrinkles are often a result.

With the aging process, the under layer has a tendency to degenerate, often causing these fibers to break into many pieces. Their supportive effectiveness is then gone, and the dermis is incapable of "standing up" by itself. In some places, the structure caves in and the outer surface falls into the crevices. These are the face's grooves, lines, and wrinkles.

The skin around the eyes and on the neck is the most likely to show these aging signs first, with the rest of the face showing the effects later.

The blood vessels, which are also in the dermis, expand with age and even may break, causing little capillary discolorations.

Protect Those Layers and Look Youthful

Remember: it is what happens in the dermis that most often creates the sense of facial aging. When damage occurs in the dermis, and happens throughout the facial area, the effects are permanent. Only cosmetic surgery can rebuild or stretch the perception of new life and youth. No matter how much care is given to the face, some structural changes will occur. But these changes can be kept to a minimum with proper care and preventive treatment. This means that paying attention to both the outer and inner layers of the skin is essential.

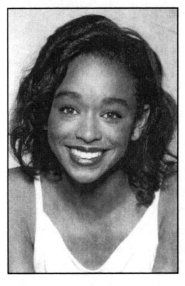

Teen Talk ... Special Things To Remember

Your remarkable skin can deal with almost anything. It adapts to stress, pain, and illness. It shrinks and stretches. It keeps out germs and bacteria – while it protects your vital organs and stores essential nutrients. It helps maintain your body temperature by preventing heat from escaping too rapidly. Your skin is your protector. Your young teenage skin is also sensitive. It works hard for you every day. So, you need to understand it if you want to look stunning.

> *Even though the outer layer of your skin receives a continuous supply of water from within, it may not be enough in all climates. Where you live, affects whether or not your skin is in danger of going dry. Use a sunscreen or moisturizing guard to protect your skin from extremely dry conditions.*

DON'TS and DO'S

Don't overeat:
Being overweight affects the condition of your skin. The stored fat accumulates peroxides, which can leave the body more open to attacks, including allergies. The fat content of foods like chips, cookies, cakes, candy, and fries is not good for your health or your skin.

Don't smoke:
Smoking cuts down on the amount of oxygen getting to the tissues, resulting in impaired circulation and a breakdown of good skin tissue. The results are dry lips, dry areas around the nose and eyes,

and a dull, ashy complexion. Nicotine is a toxic substance – a poison. Smoking is not healthy, chic, or cool!

Don't drink alcohol:
Drinking is for adults, not teens. So DON'T DRINK! Alcohol can rob your skin of vitamins and minerals – especially B, which is necessary for healthy skin. "Lite" just means a lower content of alcohol, but it's still alcohol. And remember that "coolers" so popular in the spring and summer are alcoholic beverages too.

Don't stay in the sun for long periods.
You may have heard that dark skin has more melanin than light skin. This abundance of dark pigmentation provides some protection from ultraviolet rays; but prolonged unprotected exposure to the sun can irritate even our dark skin. Unfortunately many teenagers of color go sunbathing without applying sunscreen. Because they are young, teenagers often feel that the sun will not harm them. But ultraviolet rays from the sun dry out the skin. The deeper the tan, the deeper the moisture loss. Without sufficient moisture, even creams can only do so much good. Dry skin loses its softness and suppleness, giving a dry aged look. These long or consistent short periods in the sun can cause premature lines to form between and around the eyes, toward the temple areas and around the mouth. The skin becomes blotchy and more uneven tones develop. Later on in life, the skin will lose its flexibility and develop lines and wrinkles. It may take years to see the real damage, but once done, it is just about irreversible.

Do exercise.
Proper exercise causes perspiration, which cleanses the pores and removes impurities from your system. It also increases blood flow to the surface, bringing needed nutrients to the skin. Try to get ten minutes of peak exercise a day.

Do have a full-length mirror in your bedroom.
Make sure you face the mirror nude, from all angles. This helps keep you on your diet as you see the positive changes and helps get you on a diet if you don't like the additional poundage.

Do weigh yourself regularly.
Every week, get on the same scale in the same room at the same time.

Do drink eight glasses of water daily.
Your system needs water to function properly. Remember:

o   Though water is something most of us take for granted, it is a cornerstone of good health.

o   When you are dehydrated, water improves stamina immediately.

o   Water makes up 75 percent of your body. If you don't drink water during an active day, then your thirst increases. This thirst indicates that you need water to flush your body fluids, which also keep your joints lubricated.

o   Drinking water improves chronic indigestion by keeping food moving through your digestive tract.

o   Water moisturizes the skin, cleanses the pores for a clear complexion, and flushes out poisons.

o   Don't substitute soda for water.

o   New research studies confirm that water alleviates some asthma problems by loosening mucus in the lungs and curing the common cold.

Do use a water filter:
Use a filter that draws off minerals, and traces elements from your tap water. Using filters is cheaper in the long run than buying bottled water and provides you with water that is equally tasty. Your ice cube water should be as pure as your drinking water.

Special Note

If you buy bottled water, notice that:

- Spring water usually comes from underground springs.

- Mineral water contains calcium, magnesium, iron, sodium, and other minerals.

- Sparking water is carbonated and from an underground source.

- Purified water has been distilled and filtered to remove minerals and any contaminants.

Do eat properly:
A vegetarian diet can contribute to healthy skin; but before you decide to eliminate meat and fish from your diet, consult with your physician or a dietician. If you are not a vegetarian, choose your diet with care. Eat raw, steamed vegetables, fish and chicken. Limit your intake of red meat; candy, desserts, and sugar in general, as well as tea, coffee and sodas.

Something To Think About

Many young dancers and athletes take cod liver oil, zinc, vitamins C and E, and lecithin. Before you start taking these or other vitamin supplements, such as minerals and amino acids, consult your physician or dermatologist. If you are eating properly, you may not need to include all of them in your diet.

Ask Mercedes Fleetwood:

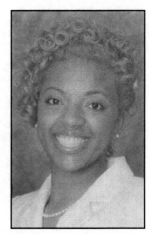

What is the most important thing that I can do to keep my skin healthy?

Keep your skin hydrated! Your skin is the largest organ in the human body and so many of us take it for granted. It gets bumped, bruised, stretched and scarred. It holds all of our organs in and blocks out germs and other unhealthy free radicals. The least we can do is give it what it needs to continue performing at its best each and every day so that we, too, can perform at our best. Hydration promotes healthy, moist, elastic skin cells, which equates to glowing, radiant, youthful skin!

I hear a lot in the news about free radicals in our environment and how bad they are for our skin. What are free radicals and what can I do to protect my skin from their harm?

Environmental factors such as pollution, radiation, cigarette smoke and herbicides can cause free radicals. Normally, your body can handle free radicals, but if antioxidants are unavailable, then they can quickly become excessive, thereby causing damage to your cells. Antioxidants can be found in vitamins C (the most abundant water-soluble antioxidant in the body) and E (the most abundant fat-soluble antioxidant in the body). The nitty gritty is: make sure you eat a well-balanced diet that includes plenty of vitamin C and vitamin E-rich fruits and veggies.

Chapter 2

How To Touch Your Face

Have you ever thought about how you touch or should touch your face? If you are like most women, you probably have not. I consider how to touch your skin so important that I make this a first "how to" section in this book. You can use all the correct products and colors, and follow the best nutrition, but still damage your face because you touch it improperly. By "touching your face," I refer to how you attend to it with your hands, such as when you clean it, apply toner, or blend on astringent, moisturizer, and other like products.

Clean Hands, Directed Movements

You should try to touch your face only when your hands are clean. Your facial skin has enough to deal with without your accidentally adding dirt and bacteria from your hands. There is a proper technique for touching your face, based on how the muscles and skin on your face are attached and how they work.

You should always use your fingers in the direction that reduces stress in a way that works with, rather than against, your facial muscles and skin. The following illustration shows the direction your fingers should move on various parts of your neck and face. When cleaning or massaging your neck, move upward with your hands or fingers to the chin line. When touching your face, use your fingertips in a circular motion, moving outward from the nose to the hairline except around the eyes.

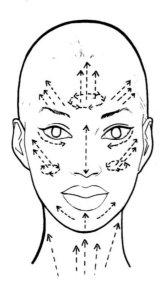

Remember, although you have five fingers, they are not equally appropriate for your face. The ring finger is most serviceable. It is your weakest finger; yes, it is even weaker than your little finger. Test it and you will see. You want to use a light touch, so use the ring finger, partially when working in the eye areas, which have the thinnest layers of epidermal skin. (That is why age lines show themselves faster and more often in these areas.)

The Eye Area

When cleansing or massaging your face around the eyes, always work from the outer temple inward toward the bridge of the nose. You should move in this direction because the facial muscles around the eyes are suspended from the temple toward the nose. Going in the opposite direction stretches the skin and muscles, and risks damage. Once damaged, there is little that can be done, other than to have injections of collagen or silicone to fill the damaged area. Most dermatologists, though, are reluctant to have black women take these injections because black skin is easily bruised and retains dark spots, either or both of which could result from such injection. I repeat: always use the ring finger under your eyes.

The Rest of the Face

Use the fingertips of your first three fingers for your cheeks, and for your forehead, move in a circular motion out to the hairline. The chin is massaged with the first three fingers of each hand, moving from the center of the chin outward with a gentle, rotating motion.

Gently Stimulate As You Touch

Whenever you touch your skin, you should try to gently massage it at the same time. The stimulation from gently slapping and massaging the face is very helpful. This form of touching causes the blood to rush upward to the surface, replenishing the skin while drawing away impurities and leaving a nice glow. Another positive is that this action reduces facial stress as well as stress throughout your body. Relaxing the facial muscles may reduce those lines in the forehead and around the mouth or prevent them from getting deeper.

If you have oily skin, however, you should stimulate your skin less often than if you have dry, because frequent massaging will bring additional oil to the surface.

Your Make-up Tools

Now that you know how to touch your face, whether you are massaging or cleansing it, you need to learn which cosmetic instruments to use when applying make-up to your face.

There are approximately seven tools that most women may use, and we will look at them one at a time: Face cloths, buff puffs, loofahs (sponges), facial tissues, cosmetic cotton balls, cosmetic swabs, and facial brushes.

Facecloths

Most people, including women, use a facecloth to wash their face and body. Unfortunately, many women do not think about the abrasive quality of their facecloth. Many cloths, after being wet from use, will dry and harden overnight, with the cloth's nap turned into a myriad of hard little bristles. When you use this cloth to scrub your face, the results —whether initially visible or not—are that you bruise and often cut the outer layer of skin, particularly around the eyes. So while cleansing you have abused your skin when your intent was just the opposite.

The guiding principal here is to show loving care to your face. Be gentle and kind. Buy and use only pure cotton facecloths because they dry softer and maintain a soft nap.

When you use a cotton facecloth, wrap it around your hand or fingers like a mitten. Work your finger, covered by the cloth, over your face as described earlier. Don't rub hard to stimulate or remove flaky skin. If you want to stimulate your face, use the massaging and slapping technique described. It will not bruise, irritate, or damage your skin or the capillaries below the surface. Don't forget: work the eye area gently, and move the cloth from the temple to the bridge of the nose. Do the forehead with a circular motion, moving outward and upward to the hairline.

Buff Puffs

Buff puffs are made of synthetic materials. They are used in washing, scrubbing, and stimulating the face. All too often, however, because of their harsh synthetic quality, the buff puff cuts or causes abrasions to the skin, resulting in a burn that may darken and become a spot. If you use a buff puff to stimulate, you must be extraordinarily careful and use it in the most gentle fashion.

If you use a buff puff, do it no more than once or twice a week, and them only with kindness and gentleness. Buff puffs should never be used if you have acne.

Loofahs

Loofahs, or luffas, are natural sponges, but they are harder and have a look of straw until they are soaked in water. There are other natural sponges, such as silk sea sponges, which are very soft and generally are used for applying make-up. When choosing a loofah, buy the softest and least abrasive one you can find. There is no doubt that, after use, your face will have a radiant glow and the look of good health, but this could be deceiving. It is possible the abrasive quality of even a soft loofah may irritate the skin in the process of stimulating the blood flow. It is best suited for using on your skin from the neck down.

Before using, always thoroughly soak the loofah in water, so it is as soft as possible. If necessary, err on the side of caution. When your face is at risk, don't use a loofah regularly; reserve it for these special occasions, and then use it gently.

Facial Tissues

There are two major "don'ts" when you think of using paper tissues on your face. The first is that you don't use tissues that contain wood pulp. Tissues applied to the face should be soft. Generally, the more expensive tissues are free of wood pulp, which, when it touches your face, can cut, scratch, or split the delicate skin mantle without your feeling or immediately knowing it. This damage can result in bruising or darkening of the healed scratch, and can even develop into a keloid (thickening of scar tissue).

The second caution is that you don't use tissues if you have excessive facial hair, skin eruptions, and so on. The fibers of the tissue may cling or get into skin openings, causing infections, discomfort, and additional problems. What is most interesting is that these concerns probably seem unnecessary because you may think they haven't happened to you. Unfortunately, the damage generally is not visible, unless you really look for it. The situation is the same as when you smoke: the injury to your body is not seen initially but by the time it is, the damage has been done.

As I consistently plead, err on the side of caution. You have everything to gain and nothing to lose. When working with tissues, use them gently and use only those free of wood fiber, when your face is smooth and free of pimples, bumps, and other blemishes.

Cotton Balls

When using cotton balls, think of them as if they were tissues. The same potential problems from using paper tissue exist for cotton balls. Buy only the pure natural-fiber cosmetic cotton balls or pads. Avoid synthetic cosmetic "cotton" balls. How can they be man-made and still be cotton? They cannot. They are damaging to your skin, so be careful; check them out.

Real cotton balls are excellent because they are sanitary. You use one, throw it away, and get another. Cotton balls are particularly good when applying toners, astringents, and fresheners, or in cleansing the delicate tissue around the eye.

Cosmetic Swabs

Your swabs should be of the best brands and of pure cotton, spun properly so that the fine cotton hairs are intact and flat on the head of the swab. This is important because loose fine cotton hairs can damage the skin, particularly when the swabs are used to clean the corners of the eyes. Properly designed pure-cotton swabs, either round or flat, are excellent for applying eye shadow, color application, and for cleansing around the nose and under the eyes. Again, as you use them in these areas, make sure that you work from the temple inward toward the bridge of the nose.

I must mention here that swabs should be used in the outer ear and not placed in the ear channel. I know this point does not relate to your face, but always when I am interviewed or on tour, women mention using swabs for their ears as well as their face. There are better ways to clean your ear channel than to place a swab in it.

Facial Brushes

I like most of the brushes on the market today, and I consider them equal in value to pure-cotton facecloths for facial use. I am particularly fond of brushes made of gentle natural or man-made fibers. Some are sponge types while others are very soft bristle form. The one type I recommend to avoid is the rubber facial brush. Dark skin bruises and marks easily, and a rubber facial brush may cause a friction burn, resulting in a bruise and discoloration.

Teen Talk ... Special Things To Remember

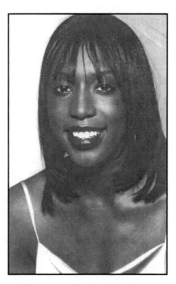

o When applying oil or cream under your eyes, gently pat it on with your ring finger.

o Before you cleanse your face, remove your eye makeup with a water-based, oil-free and fragrance-free eye make up remover, using a cotton pad and sweeping gently from the outer corner of your eye toward the bridge of your nose.

o After cleansing your face, apply toner or astringent all over your face by wiping gently with a cotton pad or ball.

o Apply both cleanser and moisturizer with fingers or an applicator. Dab the moisturizer on your nose, forehead, cheeks and chin, then massage gently in upward and outward motions.

FYI

If you're out and about and find oil seeping and spreading all over your face, try a quick fix with blotting papers.

The Best Tool For Each Job

For all of the tools mentioned, the materials you should always feel safe using on your face are your own clean fingers. You can control them better than any of these other cosmetic tools. Next best are the natural cotton facecloths and facial brush, excluding the rubber bristled ones. Don't forget: when using a facecloth, wrap it around your fingers so that you are using your fingers as though they were inside a cotton mitten. When using a facial brush, be gentle and use the same motion you would if you were using only your fingers.

Tissues, cotton balls, and swabs should all be made of pure cotton. Swabs and balls are for limited service: swabs for under eyes and in crevices around the nose; cotton balls for applying toners, astringents, and fresheners, and for cleansing. Tissues have the most limited use, mainly for cleaning or toning the face. Yet all these cosmetic tools can be serviceable if they are of fine quality and are used with care.

Don't Forget

☐ Use the fingers, and particularly the ring finger, when cleansing or touching the face.

☐ The ring finger should be used in the eye area, and the movement should be from the temple toward the bridge of the nose.

☐ Finger motion should be circular and outward to the hairline except for under the eyes.

☐ Fingers on the neck should move upward to the chin line.

☐ When stimulating the face, use the fingertips with a gentle slapping or patting motion in the directions outlined.

☐ Wrap your pure-cotton facecloth around your fingers and touch your face for cleansing as though your fingers were in a cotton mitten.

☐ The same movements you employ in using a facecloth should be used when working with a facial brush (not rubber).

Ask Mercedes Fleetwood:

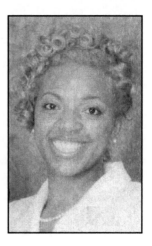

Is there such a thing as a wrong way to touch your face?

Because your skin is sensitive to the environment, your internal temperatures, hormones, and just about everything else in our world, you should treat it with love and respect at all times. Prior to touching your skin, always make sure you wash your hands with soap. Touching your face with dirty hands and nails will lead to the introduction of dirt and bacteria on your face, which can lead to unsightly rashes and bumps. When cleansing, moisturizing, and applying anything else to your face, you should apply these products in a gentle, circular motion – **Never** press down hard, use harsh pressure, rub until your skin is raw, or use your nails during any process of touching your face. This can damage the top and bottom layers of the skin and cause permanent scarring.

I have combination skin with an oily T-zone and dry patches all over. What is the healthiest and easiest regimen that I can do to maintain its youthful integrity?

If you follow these easy steps, your skin is guaranteed to be youthful, radiant, and flawless!

1. Wash your hands — If your hands are dirty you may rub bacteria or dirt onto your skin

2. Tie back your hair — this will keep the dirt and oil that is on your hair from interfering with the facial cleansing process

3. Remove your makeup — Remove your makeup with a mild makeup remover

4. Steam – this will loosen debris that may be imbedded into the skin

5. Cleanse – gently massage about a dime-size of the cleanser into your skin in a circular motion

6. Mask (optional) – apply your favorite mask to your skin in soft, circular motions. Allow it to stand on your skin for the time allotted by the mask's directions.

7. Rinse – rinse your face with lukewarm water until you feel that all of the cleanser/mask has been removed. Splash your face with cold water to temporarily shrink your pores, promote circulation, and prevent dirt from entering into your pores.

8. Dry – gently blot your face with a clean towel. Be sure to leave a small amount of water on your skin to replace some of the moisture lost during the cleansing process

9. Tone - The toner removes any traces of makeup, dirt and oil that your cleanser may have missed. it also reduces pores, eliminates oil, refines the skin, and prepares it for the moisturizer

10. Moisturize – make sure your moisturizer is appropriate to the results that you are trying to achieve. Moisturizers lock in the moisture left on your skin from the rinsing process and create a protective barrier from germs, bacteria, dirt, and free radicals, preventing them from entering into the body through the skin's pores.

Chapter 3

Your Skin Type and How to Care for It

Up to this point, I have worked with you on how to touch your face and what materials to use when cleansing, toning, and stimulating your face. You may be thinking, "That's fine, but what do I cleanse or wash my face with? Soap, creams, cleansing lotions?"

Before I can help you choose the right products to put on your face, you need to determine your skin type. You have to organize what you know about your face in order to become an effective cosmetic consumer, in terms of both value for your money and what is correct for your skin. Remember: what you put on your face *can* hurt you.

This chapter has three parts. The first helps you determine your skin type. The second discusses appropriate products for your skin type. The third applies the information conveyed in Chapter 2 to help you use the right products on your face. When you finish this chapter, you will know all the basics for using the methods described throughout the book.

Determining Your Skin Type

Many women have more than one skin type. For instance, you may have a basic skin type that is altered by outside factors. Many of you may find that there are seasonal or other reasonsyou're your skin type to change. Your skin may become dryer or oilier, or may be more sensitive than usual, based on whether it is spring/summer or fall/winter. Some women find that they have skin changes based on their menstrual period or as a result of dieting, alcohol consumption, birth-control pills, and even smoking. Additionally, drug abuse, allergies, and aging can affect your skin condition.

These effects are particularly noticeable on dark skin because it is deceptive—beautifully so—but deceptive. The amount of melanin and carotene in darker skin will often cause light to reflect off, or appear to, rather than to be absorbed, as it is on much lighter skin. If there is any perspiration on the nose or chin, the center of your face may appear shiny. This shiny quality gives the impression that the skin is oily, when actually it may not be. In fact, the skin could be dry.

A Few Simple Rules

You can look at your skin and recognize what type it is if you know how to look. Make sure you have sufficient light, meaning that it approximates daylight, and be sure the light covers your entire face. No part of your face should be in shadows. First, you will notice your T-zone. This area comprising your forehead down to the bridge of your nose, and from your nose to your chin.

If you are light or dark-skinned, you may notice light reflecting off the T-zone as you look in the mirror. Look to the left and then to the right of the T-zone, and compare how your skin looks. See if there is a different amount of light reflected on the left and right sides of the T-zone, compared to the T-zone itself.

If the sides of your face and the T-zone are the same, with clean hands touch your forehead, then the tip of your nose and your chin. If there's perspiration, wipe it away. At this point, there is more testing to do, but you probably have normal skin. If you feel oil, touch the sides of your face; if they also feel oily, then your skin is oily.

When you look at your face, note any areas that appear different, either patchy, rough, or discolored. Patchiness and roughness are often signs of dry skin; however, your face could have areas that are dry and others that are normal or oily. And this situation can change with the seasons, your health, and possible pregnancy.

Clear Your Mind and Clear Your Face

This technique for determining your skin type may seem complex, but I want you to rid yourself of all those old and untrue beliefs you may have had about your skin type. I want you to realize that skin classification requires close attention to your face as well as other conditions affecting your body. I want you to forget the notion that all you have to do is look to the T-zone or type your skin once, and the job is done forever.

For example, so many women buy the wrong products for their faces, thinking that they have sensitive skin because their faces break out. This is money wasted and keeps a skin problem unresolved.

Check Your Skin Type Twice a Year

Evaluate your skin type twice a year: once during spring/summer and once during fall/winter. But don't do it at the very beginning or end of the season. Do it a few weeks into each time, and use common sense. If the change in season is very abrupt, evaluate your face sooner; if the change is almost imperceptible do it a little later. When you change your clothes for the season, that is when to make your test. Of course, I don't mean when you change clothes to be color fashionable. I mean when you change for body comfort.

The Skin-Typing Questionnaire

Here is the easy part that helps take the guesswork and confusion out of typing your skin. I have developed ten questions, the answers to which will help you determine what kind of skin you have. The chart on the following pages shows these questions, with characteristics listed for four skin types: oily, combination, dry, and sensitive. Your answers to these ten questions can be matched to the corresponding characteristics. In some instances, there is only one description; in others, two or more situations characterize that skin type.

Questions to Determine

QUESTION	OILY
1. Before and after cleansing, can you see oil?	☐ Always
2. Does your skin feel greasy or slick?	☐ T-zone ☐ All over
3. If you bathe with deodorant soap, how does your face and body skin feel after an hour, without any type of moisturizer?	☐ Oily foreheads, eyelids, nose, and chin
4. What do your pores look like?	☐ Wide, enlarged all over
5. Do you have blackheads or whiteheads?	☐ Many ☐ Summer problems
6. Do you break out?	☐ Frequently
7. Do you peel or crack around the forehead, eyes, nose, mouth, lips, and chin?	☐ No ☐ Summer ☐ Occasionally in winter, especially around nose and mouth
8. Does your skin look tight, smooth, and ashen?	☐ Rarely
9. Does your cleanser and moisturizer sit on top of your skin or disappear immediately into it?	☐ Never disappears
10. How do you react to sun?	☐ Rarely burn, good tan

Your Skin Type

COMBINATION	DRY	SENSITIVE
☐ Sometimes: ☐ Oily in spring/summer Dry in fall/winter	☐ Rarely	☐ Sometimes: ☐ Summer problems
☐ T-zone	☐ T-zone ☐ Summer	☐ T-zone ☐ Sometimes
☐ Slightly dry-looking in appearance and feel Jawline and around eyes in fall/winter	☐ Taut, tight, and dry in feeling and appearance with ashen dull cast	☐ Tight and shiny T-zone after first half-hour ☐ Sometimes in winter
☐ Enlarged in T-zone, especially on nose, cheek, and chin	☐ Almost invisible, fine pores	☐ Noticeable in T-zone, fine elsewhere
☐ T-zone problems Cheeks	☐ Few ☐ Summer problems	☐ Occasionally
☐ Occasionally	☐ Rarely ☐ Few in summer	☐ Always ☐ Rashes and patches
☐ Occasionally	☐ Frequently ☐ Around eyes, forehead, mouth, lips, and chin, especially in winter	☐ Occasionally ☐ Around eyes and nose
☐ Sometimes ☐ Winter	☐ Frequently, on forehead, cheeks, jawline, and chin	☐ Rarely
☐ Sometimes disappears	☐ Always disappears immediately	☐ Sometimes disappears
☐ Slow burn, especially in summer	☐ Burn easily without moisture protection	☐ Burn easily without moisture protection

Analyzing Your Skin Type

We classify your skin to help you buy products that are designed for your basic skin type. These products cannot be tailored to your exact skin, however. It is like fashion designing. If you have a personal fashion designer, he or she can tailor a pattern and change it as your body changes, in order to produce clothes exactly for your body. However, when you go to the department store, no matter how upscale it is, you must choose an item from "the rack." It must be altered to fit you, and those altered measurements are made only in a few places. In cosmetics, there are no after-purchase refinements or tailoring. You take the product from "the rack" and use it as recommended by the beauty adviser, based on the skin-type information you have provided.

In recent times, the cosmetics and beauty industry has done an excellent and thoughtful job of researching skin types. The products they offer cover a wide enough range both to properly address your skin's needs and to enhance it while maintaining its health. You can analyze your skin type closely enough to achieve proper product selection. By reviewing the skin-type analysis chart you can use your answers to the skin-typing questions to determine your actual skin type. Based on which column most of your answers fall into, you will know your basic skin type.

Your Skin-Care Regimen

Now that you have determined your skin type, you can think in terms of proper facial care. When I mention "facial care," be aware that you can only address the epidermis. There are no products that penetrate deeper. Remember: proper external care and proper nutrition are two keys to healthy, beautiful skin. If you add the third key—stress reduction—you not only will have healthy, beautiful skin but it will have fewer lines and your life expectancy will be extended.

Start now with a proper skin-care program. There are three basic steps to any quality skin regimen: cleanse, tone, moisturize. These are followed by a maintenance step, a special beauty procedure.

Cleanse

Select a cleanser that meets the needs of your type skin, then relax your face, massaging it as described in Chapter 2. See the following illustration. The cleanser will help remove the outer cells layer and the impurities imbedded in your pores. (Clogged pores are a major reason for skin eruptions or blackheads.) The cleanser should clean deep but gently.

When choosing a cleanser for use during the summer, women with oily and combination skin should think in terms of lightweight or light-textured products such as water-soluble lotions and gels. These clean gently and have less detergent, and less of a drying effect on the skin. In the winter, women with dry skin might look to creams and rich emollients.

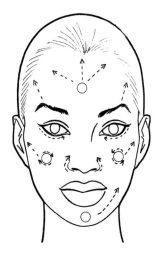

Step 1.
Cleanse, following the illustrated direction of application

Try more than one of these products for your skin type, because each will be a little different. When you find the cleanser you like best, stay with it until you type your skin again, when there might be a need for a change, or if your skin reacts to the product. Remember, though that when your skin reacts, it may not be to the cleanser. First look to your diet, drinking habits, menstrual period, oral contraception, or possible pregnancy. If these are all eliminated as the cause, look to stress. When it, too, is determined not to be the cause, look at the products you are using. But generally, if properly chosen, your cleanser will not be the cause. Of all products, skin cleansers are the most researched and tested.

Tone

Products used for toning the skin, which you may have heard of or have even used yourself, are astringents, skin fresheners, refining lotions, and clarifying lotions. A toner rinses off any cleanser or soap film on the face. But in our regimen it does even more than that. Its other purpose is to prepare your skin to receive a moisturizer. And it has yet another purpose. Do you remember that in Chapter 1 I mentioned the pH factor and the belief that the skin's natural acidity helps protect it from bacterial infection? A toner restores the pH to a proper level and corrects the balance of oil and water on the skin's surface.

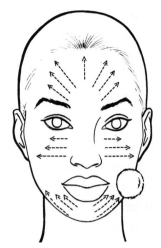

Step 2.
Apply toner, following illustrated direction of application.

A toner is particularly important for those women with oily, dry, or sensitive skin, for it will attend to their skin's balance needs. Look at the Beauty Resource Guide in the appendix and choose a toner suited to your skin type. Then apply it as shown in the following illustration.

Moisturize

Moisturizers do different things for different skin types. However, they will do the following for all skin types: become a sealer to hold skin moisture in (emollients) and draw moisture from the air to the skin to help keep it lubricated (humectant). If your skin is dry, then your moisturizer will lubricate and protect your face with an oil based mixture which adds necessary oil. If your skin is oily, then your moisturizer will be oil-free, for your skin has all the oil it needs. The moisture will also be water-based, fragrance-free, and dermatologically tested since such skin has a tendency to be sensitive. Apply the moisturizer as shown in the following illustration.

A moisturizer is a liquid or cream with two critical ingredients: a humectant and emollients. A humectant attracts and absorbs moisture in and on the surface of the skin as long as possible. They are either oil or non-oil substances in accordance with whether you have dry skin (oil-based) or oily skin (non-oil-based).

If you have combination skin, consider the time of the year and the condition of your body. If it's winter and your skin is dry in places (for example, on your jaw or chin), use a moisturizer for dry skin in those areas and one for normal skin elsewhere. If it's summer and your T-zone is oily, concentrate on a moisturizer for oily skin.

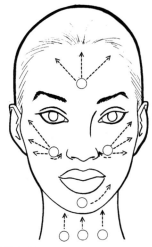

Step 3.
Apply moisturizer with fingers or applicator in the direction illustrated.

All too often, women who have dry skin apply mineral oil, petroleum jelly, or cocoa butter to the eye area. This suffocates the tissue around the eyes; it cannot breathe, and it swells and gets puffy. This is exactly what you don't want. Always use a specially formulated eye oil—a lightweight, refined oil cream for this delicate area. Massage the cream in, gently patting it on with your ring finger and working from the temple down to the nose. For oily-skinned women, I recommend oil-free eye preparations to lubricate this area.

A Special Beauty Step

The special beauty step is a maintenance one. Once or twice a week, based on your skin type, you should use an exfoliating lotion, cream, or gel. These exfoliates are for deep cleansing. They reach deeper into the epidermis than can your daily cleanser.

During general cleansing each day and evening, often specific types of problem skin—for example, very dry or very oily skin—require a super cleansing. Based on the season of year and your skin type, I suggest that you indulge in weekly deep cleansing and treatment. By "deep cleansing" I mean to cleanse, tone, exfoliate or mask, and so on.

If, for example, you have dry skin and it is wintertime, use a mask in spots, so as to deal exclusively with the problem area and leave the rest of your face alone. If you have oily skin and it is summertime, use an exfoliate and/or a deep-pore cleansing mask to rid your skin of dead cells and to unclog your pores.

When choosing a cleanser, make sure the ingredients are not harmful or abrasive to the skin. Some general cleaners contain grains which act as a mild exfoliate and skin stimulator. Often, the grains remove the outer layer of skin. But when the grains are chips of shells or nuts, they often have pointed, sharp edges that can scrape, split, and damage the outer layer of facial skin. Natural grains, unlike shells and nuts, are rounded and will not cut or cause such damage; they dissolve as you gently massage and scrub.

You may be thinking about one consideration I haven't yet mentioned: the eye area. This is the most delicate area, with the thinnest and fewest layers of skin. When cleansing, use the mildest nonabrasive cleansers and remember to use your fingers gently in this area and to move them from the temple toward the bridge of your nose.

Now that we have outlined the general skin-care regimen, let's get specific in terms of coupling your skin type with your specific skin-care regimen.

The Oily Skin Classification

If your skin is normal to oily, there is a basic regimen to help you balance and control the oil. It's important that you drink eight glasses of water a day to flush your system of internal impurities and excess oil. Your oily skin systematically produces too much oil, day and night. If the surface sebum (sebaceous oil) is not removed at least twice a day, your skin mantle collects oil, perspiration, bacteria, and impurities that will cause problems—for example, clogged pores, blackheads, and acne.

Usually, oily skin is noticeably uneven in skin tone, light in the center of the face (T-zone), and slightly dark at the temples, outer cheeks, lower jawline, and chin. It is plagued with constant flare-ups and breakouts. Oily skin has visibly wide pores and a greasy, slick feeling. It can even appear dull.

A clean face is your goal. Oily skin must be washed at least once during the day and again before retiring. (The desired cleansing is at least three times a day, reapplying fresh make-up when convenient.) Your oily skin is not a problem when you know what to do. But you must plan your time and take care to meet your skin's requirements.

Day Care

PRODUCTS TO USE	PRODUCT DIRECTIONS
Step 1. Cleanse Use lotion and liquid soap detergents formulated for oily skin. Nondeodorant soap bar (facial soap) also is recommended for oily skin. Use oil-free water-based products.	Use tepid (lukewarm) water to rinse your skin. I do not recommend a cream cleanser on oily skin during the spring/ summer months in any region. Water- based cleansing lotions are fine if without mineral oil. (Lotion cleansers are excellent for removing stale make-up prior to deep-pore cleansing.) Note: Acne oily skin is a medical problem and requires the attention of a dermatologist. Ask your dermatologist about products before you purchase. Gentle facial brushes are excellent but scrubs are best to help clean clogged pores. A natural fiber puff and non rubber cleansing brushes are recommended.
Step 2. Tone Use a fragrance-free astringent and formula for oily skin. Skin fresheners and clarifying lotions formulated for oily skin are excellent for fall/winter.	Use lavishly; apply with cotton ball or pad and wipe until clean. Avoid the eye area. Also, don't use an astringent that has resorcinol, a skin-darkening agent.
Step 3. Moisturize Use water-based, oil- and fragrance-free formulas for oily skin only.	Light moisturizers are water-holding agents that protect, retain moisture, and shield against the environment. Place 4 dots of moisture lotion at the forehead, cheeks, and chin and massage into skin. No residue or tacky feeling should exist.
For lips, a mineral-oil lip moisturizer is excellent. No oil-producing glands exist on top or bottom lips, so mineral oil can seal in and protect dry tissue against the environment. Oily skin types can have dry lips during all seasons.	Apply a cocoa butter, camphor, beeswax, lanolin, or petrolatum lip moisturizer directly from the tube or pat on your lips. This formula is for lips only, and is not appropriate for the facial area ever!

Evening Care

PRODUCT TO USE	PRODUCT DIRECTIONS
Step 1. Cleanse Step 2. Tone Step 3. Moisturize	Same as for day care
Special Night Care: Use a waster-based oil- and fragrance- free eye make-up remover.	Use product with a cotton ball or cotton eye pad to remove eye make-up. Rinse with tepid water to remove all traces. Sweep in gently with your ring finger from the outer corner of each eye toward the bridge of the nose.
Eye Treatment: Use formula for oily skin.	
Neck treatment: Cleanse, tone, moisturize, and apply night cream or anti-aging preparation.	Massage the formula into skin at the neck and throat area. See face chart, Chapter 2.

Weekly Care

PRODUCT TO USE	PRODUCT DIRECTIONS
Use a deep-pore exfoliate or scrub formulated for oily skin. Clay mask with conditioning properties is best for oily skin, especially in spring and summer, if fragrance-free.	Deep-pore cleansing dislodges imbedded dirt in the pores and removes the outer layer of skin-dulling dead cells. Cleansing grains are great, but avoid formulas with sharp particles, since they scratch and scar delicate skin tissue.

Your goal is oil control. You don't want to deplete the skin's natural oil, but you do want to kill the shine. An advantage to oily skin is that women of color with oily skin appear to age less and at a slower rate, owing to the oily deposits deep in the layers of the dermis.

Here are some do's and don'ts for women with oily skin:

Do's

- ❑ Do drink eight glasses of water daily.
- ❑ Do use only water-based, oil-free, fragrance-free products.
- ❑ Do use astringents as often as you can—day and night as well as weekly.
- ❑ Do use a clay mask at least twice weekly, spring/summer, and once a week in fall/winter.
- ❑ Do avoid fatty foods.

Don'ts

- ❑ Don't use oil-based creams, lotions, or soaps.
- ❑ Don't use acne-medicated cleansing pads as an astringent. You'll dry out areas around the eyes, temples, nose, and chin.
- ❑ Don't use abrasive cleansing pads, buff puffs, or loofahs on your face frequently.
- ❑ Don't use PURE alcohol, witch hazel, hydrogen peroxide, or concentrated lemon juice as an astringent.

The Dry Skin Classification

If your skin is normal to dry, there is a basic regimen to help you maintain a balance between moisture and oil. It's important that you drink six to eight glasses of water a day to restore the body's moisture and to flush your system of impurities. You should also know that dry skin requires serious attention.

Coating and pore-sealing oils—such as baby oil, mineral oil, and petroleum products—do not condition or relieve rough, patchy, flaking, and sometimes uncomfortably itchy skin. The ashen skin will disappear when these coating and sealing oils are applied, but they clog the pores and allow particles from the environment to stick to the skin.

Dry skin can look dull and gray or ashen, be sensitive, and often be painful. Its fine pores can clog and break out. The problem areas are the forehead, lower cheeks, jawline, and chin. A dry, peeling nose can have fine dirt imbedded as blackheads and whiteheads on the side and tip, invisible and unnoticeable but sensitive to the touch. Dry skin reacts to extreme cold and hot temperatures, and suffers from a lack of both internal and surface moisture (dehydration) as well as from inadequate production of surface oil (sebum). Dry skin ages faster than oily or combination skin. The result can be premature wrinkles and crepey-looking lines around the eyes and mouth.

Day Care

PRODUCT TO USE	PRODUCT DIRECTIONS
Step 1. Cleanse Select a dry-skin oil cleanser if your skin is extremely dry, a rich creamy formula if your skin is moderately dry, and, if you are a soap-and-water person, a nondeodorant formula with rich emollients and conditioners designed for dry skin.	Tissue or rinse off. Massage gently, always moving upward and outward; see face chart in Chapter 2. Rinse with tepid water until your face is absolutely clean.
Step 2. Tone Use a non-alcohol toner for extremely dry skin or a low-alcohol toner for moderately dry skin.	Apply with a cotton ball or pad and wipe until all traces of surface impurities are gone.
Step 3. Moisturize Select a rich dry-skin emollient with moisturizers and conditioners specifically for dry skin. I prefer the fragrance-free tested formulas.	Smooth in gently from the base of your neck, massaging from the throat area upward to the hairline.
Your lips suffer in the winter. Use a mineral-oil lip preparation to trap and seal moisture on your lips. Medicated formulas relieve cracked, peeling, bleeding, and splitting.	Gently smooth in the penetrating emollient. Do not apply this formula to your face.

Evening Care

PRODUCT TO USE	PRODUCT DIRECTIONS
Step 1. Cleanse Step 2. Tone Step 3. Moisturize	Same as for day care.
Special Night Care: Use a no-tear, fragrance-free, derma-tologically tested make-up remover.	Use product with a cotton ball or cotton pad to remove eye make-up. Rinse with tepid water to remove all traces.
Eye Treatment: use a rich light-tex-tured emollient.	Sweep in gently with your ring finger from the outer corner of each eye toward the bridge of the nose.
Anti-aging treatment: use a night cream or anti-aging cell-renewal for-mula for your extremely dry, line- and wrinkle- prone skin. Mature dry skin may require a special firming cream or lotion to help soften and smooth the skin and restore a healthy glow.	Massage formula into skin on neck, throat, face, ears, and at hairline.

Weekly Care

PRODUCT TO USE	PRODUCT DIRECTIONS
Use a moisturizing cream to slough and peel off dry skin. (If you have thick facial hair, the peel-off type is not recommended.) Avoid clay or drawing formulas because they remove too much natural oil and moisture.	Apply a thin film of moisturizer over extremely dry skin before applying a gel peel-off mask. Cream the mask with healing conditioners—e.g., Aloe Vera.

Your goal is to replenish and maintain the balance of water and oil on your delicate skin surface. You want to rid the skin of dulling dead facial cells and impurities.

You must take every preventive step to lubricate and hold moisture on your skin. Harsh winter and summer air robs your skin of its natural moisture and oil. You can retard the deepening and lining of your face with proper care and with moisture-conditioning formulas that penetrate the layers of the epidermis.

Here are some do's and don'ts for women with dry skin:

Do's

- ❑ Do drink eight glasses of water daily.
- ❑ Do use only oil-based, moisture-conditioning, dermatologically tested products.
- ❑ Do use a cream mask for very dry skin.
- ❑ Do ventilate your daytime and evening rooms. Humidifiers are an excellent way to control moisture.
- ❑ Do use spot facial masks during summer and winter, applying them to problem areas only.

Don'ts

- ❑ Don't use astringents formulated for oily and combination skin.
- ❑ Don't use abrasive, exfoliating granular-based masks.
- ❑ Don't use deodorant-type soaps on your face. From the neck down, deodorant soaps are fine.
- ❑ Don't use petroleum jelly, cocoa butter, mineral oil, or baby oil as a facial moisturizer, especially if you are going to wear a cream or liquid-cream make-up foundation. Cocoa butter and petroleum by-products are excellent for the lower body parts, however.

The Combination Skin Classification

Your skin may be oily, dry, or sensitive in different areas, and it requires special attention in both summer and winter. There is a basic regimen you should follow to maintain a balance between moisture and oil. It's important that you drink eight glasses of water a day to flush your system of internal impurities and to restore the balance of water and oil on the surface of the skin.

When in balance, a combination skin can actually be normal. But seasonal conditions can affect combination skin to the point where it may be normal during one season and dry or oily during another. Additionally, stress, a dramatic weight loss or gain, dietary food changes, an irregular menstrual cycle, and aging can disturb the natural balance of acidity, moisture, oil, and dryness.

Skin eruptions, breakouts and patchy rashes can sometimes occur on your forehead, cheeks, and chin. Your pores are fine around the hairline, temples, chin, and jawline but visible in the T-zone. Your skin can be part oily and part dry at the same time, so you must select appropriate treatment products for areas of your face and time of year.

Day Care

PRODUCT TO USE	PRODUCT DIRECTIONS
Step 1. Cleanse Use a liquid soap with mild detergent and facial shampoo properties. There are water-based lotions and nondrying facial cleansing soap bars designed for normal to combination skin.	Splash on water and rinse thoroughly with tepid water. Use the face chart in Chapter 2 for proper movement directions as you massage.
Step 2. Tone Use an astringent for oily zones in summer. Use a skin freshener for normal to dry zones in winter.	Dampen a cotton ball or pad and wipe until ball or pad is absolutely clean.
Step 3. Moisturize Use a lotion or lightweight soufflé-type moisturizer.	For summer oiliness, apply oil-free moisturizer all over, from neck to forehead. For winter dryness, apply soufflé-type moisturizer cream. Apply moisturizer with fingers or applicator in the direction illustrated on page .
For lips in winter use a moisturizer on both lips.	Apply directly from tube or pat on.

Evening Care

PRODUCT TO USE	PRODUCT DIRECTIONS
Step 1. Cleanse Step 2. Tone Step 3. Moisturize	Same as for day care.
Special Night Care: Use eye make-up remover for combination-type skin.	Use product with a cotton ball or cotton pad to remove eye make-up. Rinse with tepid water to remove all traces.
Eye treatment: use formulas appropriate for dry and oily eye zones.	Using the ring finger, gently apply eye preparation over and under the eye.

Weekly Care

PRODUCT TO USE	PRODUCT DIRECTIONS
Anti-aging treatment: use cell-renewal firming lotions or creams and night creams designed for dry and oily skin.	A few drops of this firming formula is applied to the problem aging areas.
Problem areas: use a clay mask for oily areas. A creamy mask with soft grains helps draw out toxins, heals, and firms and alleviates whiteheads and blackheads.	Spot-mask the oily areas twice a month in the summer and once a month in the winter for 6-10 minutes. Avoid applying clay mask to dry areas of the face.

Your goals are to treat, care for, and maintain your normal to combination skin. Summer emphasis is on the oily zones and winter efforts are on healing and conditioning the dry areas. Weekly deep-pore cleansing is important.

Here are some do's and don'ts for women with combination skin:

Do's

❑ Do drink eight glasses of water daily.

❑ Do use oil-free products that are light in texture for the summer season.

❑ Do choose skin fresheners and toners formulated for normal and combination skin, based on the season.

❑ Do use products formulated and tested for normal and combination-type skin.

Don'ts

❑ Don't use the same product year-round. Your skin type changes dramatically. Observe your skin and note the oily and dry areas.

❑ Don't use abrasive cosmetic tools over the entire face, especially in the winter months.

The Sensitive Skin Classification

If your skin is sensitive, there is a basic regimen that will calm, balance, and alleviate discomfort. It's important that you drink eight glasses of water daily to rid your body of external impurities. Use fragrance- and oil-free products. Hypoallergenic or dermatologically tested products are applicable.

Your skin type has less tolerance of chemical substances and reacts to bad dietary habits, stress, hormonal changes, allergies, trauma, and impurities in the environment. It tends to be more dry in certain areas and may have frequent skin eruptions. Your skin may bruise easily and dark spots may be the result. Cosmetics companies have made excellent efforts to meet your sensitive skin-care needs, with products that are dermatologically tested to heal, soothe, and relieve your skin conditions and to improve your skin texture.

I recommend that you consult a dermatologist for treating extreme or severe sensitive skin conditions. And have a cosmetologist or beauty advisor do a patch test before you purchase a new product; you might even take a sample of that product to your dermatologist.

Day Care

PRODUCT TO USE	PRODUCT DIRECTIONS
Step 1. Cleanse In summer, use a lotion, liquid soap, or facial soap bar. In winter, use a liquid cream or cream formula that is fragrance- and oil-free. Use products tested for dark-toned sensitive skin.	Massage liquid facial shampoo and lotion gently with your fingertips, using the face chart in Chapter 2. Rinse thoroughly. Tissue off or rinse off water-soluble creams.
Note: Do not squeeze acne pimples, or dark scarring may occur. Do not use harsh cleansers or scrubs. Do not aggravate overactive oil glands or eruptions. Preparations are on the market to correct young people's and adult acne. See a dermatologist.	

PRODUCT TO USE	PRODUCT DIRECTIONS
Step 2. Tone Use a skin freshener designed for dark-toned sensitive skin, with low or no alcohol or resorcinol. Skin fresheners fight bacteria, balance the oil and moisture levels on your skin, and refine the pores.	Wipe the entire face, avoiding eye zones, until a cotton pad or ball is absolutely clean.
Step 3. Moisturize Use fragrance-free and oil-free treated lotions, or light, creamy soufflé-type moisturizers, that are formulated for dark-toned sensitive skin after liquid facial soap shampoos and toners. Fragrance- and oil-free moisturizers are water-holding agents to protect, condition, and smooth surface tissue.	In summer your skin does not need a coating or sealing of moisturizer. In winter apply a light film of cream.

Evening Care

PRODUCT TO USE	PRODUCT DIRECTIONS
Step 1. Cleanse Step 2. Tone Step 3. Moisture	Same as for day care.
Special Night Care: Use a no-tear, fragrance-free, hypoallergenic, tested eye make-up remover.	Use product with a cotton ball or cotton pad to remove eye make-up. Rinse with tepid water to remove all traces.
Eye treatment: use a cream designed for dry and sensitive skin.	Sweep in from the outer corner of each eye, toward the bridge of the nose, gently applying the cream with your ring finger.
Anti-aging treatment: use a cell-renewal preparation for sensitive skin.	Massage formula into skin on neck, throat, face, and at hairline.

Weekly Care

PRODUCT TO USE	PRODUCT DIRECTIONS
Problem areas: use a clay or drawing-formula mask to lift blackheads and draw out toxins and other impurities. Use peel-off or moisture-conditioning masks to clean deep, lifting away accumulated dead cells.	In summer, spot-mask problem oily areas only. (Not recommended for dry areas.) In winter, spot-mask on dry skin zones only.

Your goal is to be as gentle as possible with your skin. Attend to break-outs or acne eruptions immediately. Your hands and fingertips carry microorganisms that breed on dirt, stale make-up, and polluted oil, so keep hands and fingers off your face.

You must select a treatment system from one cosmetics company. Do not mix treatment products (for example, don't combine cleanser from **X**, toner from **Y**, and moisturizer from **Z**). Fragrance- and oil-free, water-based products that have been tested by dermatologists are recommended.

Here are some do's and don'ts for women with sensitive skin:

Do's

- ❑ Do drink eight glasses of water daily.
- ❑ Do use acne-cleansing pads without resorcinol, which is a darkening agent.
- ❑ Do stay calm and learn to relax to help chase skin problems away.
- ❑ Do develop better dietary habits. What you put in your body affects your skin.
- ❑ Do use special astringent or skin fresheners formulated for sensitive skin.
- ❑ Do keep your face's dry zones in check.

Don'ts

- ❑ Don't use astringents designed for oily skin on dry zones of your face.

- ❑ Don't eat a lot of dairy products, salty and oily foods, or sugar-filled products including chocolates.

Now you know your skin type and have a regimen for daily care. You should, however, take into account the season—spring/summer or fall/winter—when you answer the skin-typing questionnaire. And don't forget to ask yourself if there are any special changes going on: Are you dieting? Do you have your period? Been doing a "lot of partying?" I am sure you know this already, for I mentioned it early on, but it's worth repeating. Since the germinating layer of your skin is fed through your blood system, what you eat and what gets into your blood system has a noticeable effect on your face.

Teen Talk...Special Things To Remember

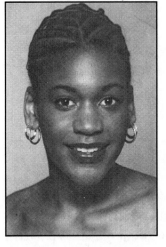

The Basics of a Flawless Complexion

Using soaps on your face is not recommended because most soap bars are highly alkaline and usually the skin will become dry, irritated, patchy, blotchy and discolored.

Skip petroleum jelly. Many teens think of petroleum jelly as a facial "de-asher"; meaning from the neck down, it becomes the all-purpose "ash-killer". Your skin may look like it's taking on a healthy sheen, but you're really doing more harm than good.

The basic steps to your quality skincare regimen are very simple:

1. Cleanse with a "facial cleanser".

2. Tone with a skin freshener or toner.

3. Moisturize with a moisturizer, made especially for your skin type (dry, oily or normal).

Teen Tip:

For a healthy complexion, you should just make sure you use the right stuff on your skin. Test the product on a small spot before using it all over your face. If you're not sure what to buy, ask for assistance at the cosmetic counter or check with your dermatologist.

Ask Mercedes Fleetwood:

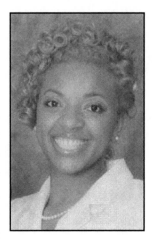

My skin is easily irritated and I often break out in a fine rash. What can I do about it?

I recommend exfoliating gently with a sugar scrub because the sodium in salt scrubs tends to further inflame irritation-prone skin. When exfoliating any body part, you should always massage gently in circular motions. We have a tendency to be impatient and somehow we believe that the harder we work, the faster we will see results. This is a false-ism when it comes to skin care! Our skin is not a block of wood and the exfoliating scrub is not coarse sand paper; rather, our skin is a gentle organ that is sensitive to touch and pressure, and it should be respected as such. Do NOT disrespect your skin! When choosing a moisturizer, look for one that is rich in alpha-hydroxy-acids (AHA's) or lactic acid as they help dissolve the keratin and build-up of excess skin cells. The combination of both frequent exfoliation and a moisturizer rich in AHAs will have your skin supple and smooth.

Ageless Beauty

Chapter 4

Facial Hair, Blemishes, and Other Facial Conditions

In this chapter I explain why there are certain skin features such as facial hair, freckles, pimples and blemishes, blackheads and whiteheads, age spots, and so on. If you understand what causes these conditions and know how to cover or remove them effectively and safely, then you will feel better about your face and about your self.

Removing Facial Hair

Hair, particularly facial hair, is a condition many women must address, especially women if color. It is not these women necessarily have more facial or body hair, but the problem has to be approached differently. When facial hair is a problem—for example, when hair bumps detract from one's appearance or interfere with make-up application, it is an issue to be addressed.

Facial Waxing

Areas of concern are usually the facial hair at the temples, hair at the jawline moving back toward the ear lobe, and hair on the upper lip or chin. More women than you might realize have thick hair growing above their upper lip or on the base of their chin. If you want clear skin, then such hair must be removed, especially if you wish your make-up to have a clear, smooth appearance.

Most white women, especially Nordic women, are fair-skinned and have blonde or sandy-colored hair. They can readily bleach these facial hairs and the hairs appear to fade to become translucent. For most black women, bleaching is not an option. The bleached hair stands out prominently against your dark skin. The only recourse is to have this facial hair professionally removed by waxing. Waxing is a hair removal technique that involves applying a paste of warm wax to the hair surface. The wax is allowed to dry, then it is stripped away. As it is stripped away, so is the hair, leaving the skin beneath smooth. It is painless, and the method can keep the area free of hair for from three to six weeks. Another option is to purchase on over-the-counter hair-removing wax product from a drugstore chain or department store. You can use these products at home, and while the process takes time, you will save money. The home method keeps hairs off for nearly six weeks.

Electrolysis and Depilatrom

Hair can be removed permanently through electrolysis or depilatrom. Sometimes you may experience a degree of sensitivity from depilatrom, but this doesn't last long. Electrolysis, however, can be very costly, since you pay by the number of hairs removed.

Some dermatologists do not recommend electrolysis for women of color because many develop scarring around the pores. These areas are damaged and become unsightly after the hairs have been pulled through or by them. Some women build up such scar tissue around the pores that they develop keloids (bumps composed of scar tissue). Dark skin, although multi-layered, is susceptible to scarring—certainly more so than light skin. Make sure you have a competent electrolysis technician who understands dark skin.

There are new gadgets that remove hair electronically, so you can do the procedure at home yourself. Usually such items are sold in the beauty-appliance section of the retail cosmetics outlet or cosmetics counter in better drugstores.

Unruly Eyebrows

Another area of hair growth on the face is the eyebrows. Knowing the technique of shaping the eyebrows is important. A woman is considered lucky if she has eyebrow hairs that lay flat and the eyebrows that are well shaped to complement her eyes. However, most women are not so lucky, and they have to have some hairs removed to get a nice look. Many women prefer not to wear a great deal of eye shadow, but if they do, bushy or unruly hairs springing through the eye shadow and highlighter is unsightly. Others have eyebrow hairs removed because they don't like the way their eyebrows look and can't find a way to manage them. For example, bushy or heavy and coarse eyebrows may require some plucking.

I find it most unattractive when a woman shaves off her eyebrows and then uses an eyebrow pencil to draw in a line. This gives the face a severe look. Why shave the eyebrow off and then put a new one on, instead of properly shaping or filling in your existing eyebrow?

Nothing is more unsightly than a dramatic, overplucked eyebrow, either. The problem that this may cause—beyond unsightliness—is that when you continually pluck hairs in certain spots, you pull out some of the roots and the hairs will never grow back. Thus you are left with a patchy-looking brow.

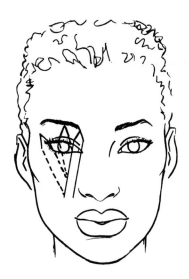

To determine the best length and thickness of your brow, hold the pencil to each nostril and straight up along the nose to the eyebrow. Where it touches the eyebrow is where the brow should begin. Hair between the eyebrows should be removed. Position the pencil vertically over the center of your eye to the beginning of the arch. When you position the pencil from the nose to the outer edge of the eye, you determine the endpoint of the brow and arch.

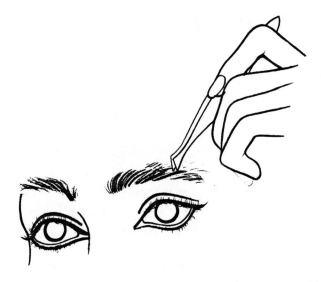

Look in the mirror and honestly assess the length and thickness of your brows. If they are bushy and are overpowering your face, then you should remove some hairs. If your eyebrows are too thick and spotty with nicks, then you should shape the brow to complement a natural eyeline. With a brow pencil, you can stroke in between the spaces, filling and shaping the brow. The drawn-on pencil is out of fashion; instead, start from the center of the eye and go upward to the temple, removing from eight to ten hairs.

Tweeze the stray hairs underneath your brow, also. The ideal eyebrow arch is smooth and soft—often referred to as a moon shape. Shape your eyebrow with the peak at the top of your pencil in the center of the brow.

Body Hair

You may want to remove hair from your legs, around the neck, and under your arms. Waxing can rid these areas of unwanted hair. There are also depilatories sold in any beauty department that easily whisks away the hair. Let the depilatory set for a few moments and then wipe or rinse hair off with water. Always apply a moisturizer after removing hair from either the face or lower body parts.

Skin Problems

Let's look at the skin "problems" most black women ask me about. Remember, even if you avoid the "don'ts" and do the "do's" in Chapter 3, you may still have skin problems.

Breaking Out

There is no one, specific cause for "breaking out," but it can almost always be stopped or controlled. No matter what the cause, good, regular skin care can help. A healthy regimen plus internal medicine can cure most, if not all, incidents of breaking out and prevent their recurrence.

The type, form, and amount of medicine should be determined by a physician. Obviously, you need not go to the doctor for every blemish. But when you have a blemish that doesn't go away and it bothers you, seek medical advise. Yes, even acne is a condition worthy of a doctor's visit. The person at the cosmetics counter is a beauty adviser, not a physician, even if he or she is a licensed cosmetologist.

The Pill Is Not a Skin Enhancer

Many women have asked me about taking birth-control pills to clear up their skin problems. At this time there is no consensus on the pill's effectiveness in treating skin problems. Research has been done in this area, but at least 25 percent of those studied have seen their skin worsen, and the largest group studied saw no change in skin condition at all. The estrogen in birth-control pills is sometimes used as a skin treatment, but I am opposed to using the pill that way. There are possible side effects from birth-control pills, among them an increase in skin pigmentation and, for some women, the skin gets mottled and darkish.

Menses and Skin Eruptions

Yes, there is an established relationship between your periods and facial eruptions or breakouts. But preventive medication is available. Don't forget, though, that careful cleansing before, during, and after your period definitely helps.

Blemishes

Blemishes are skin faults—for example, blackheads, whiteheads, and pimples. When you see a blackhead, do you probe and squeeze it? You should not. Squeezing a blackhead can damage the surrounding areas, and you can spread the infection to below the surface, causing other places on your face to erupt. The best way to remove or eliminate blackheads is to keep your skin clean. Remember, you can't have a blackhead without a clogged, oily pore. Therefore, the best approach is super cleanliness—morning and night, and sometimes in between.

The whitehead is so named because the head of the eruption is whitish in color. There are stubborn cases when whiteheads persist, and you should see a doctor or dermatologist, who'll treat it with a miniature scalpel or electric needle. Whiteheads found around the eye (milia) are generally believes to be caused by abrasions or small cuts.

Blotches

To avoid blotches, avoid excessive sunlight. Limit the amount of ultraviolet light that hits your face by using a sunblock, either all over the face or on just the mottled area. Actually, sunblock is a great base for make-up.

If mottled, darkish spots already exist on your face, it is possible to have then removed through dermabrasion—the wearing down of the skin layers, until there is clear skin. There are also abrasive scrubs and bleaching creams that can be used directly on the affected area, which help work off the dead, darkened skin.

Wrinkles and Sagging Skin

Wrinkles and sagging skin are due to a breakdown of the skin's collagen, connective tissue, which maintains the skin's elasticity and tightness. Proper skin care not only keeps your skin clear and free of blemishes, but also retards the breaking down of the skin's collagen, reducing wrinkles and sagging skin. Therefore, it is critical that you maintain an adequate collagen level. This can easily be attained by consuming adequate amounts of vitamin C daily. A natural source of vitamin C is rosehips. A rich natural source of vitamins, rosehips contain twenty to forty times more vitamin C than oranges. They also have twenty-five times more vitamin A, 28 percent more calcium, and 25 percent more iron than oranges. Rosehips are extremely rich in Bioflavonoids—co-factors in the vitamin C complex. But whatever you take—natural foods or vitamins—make vitamin C one of your staples, for it is a most important health and facial rejuvenation vitamin.

By utilizing these nutritional tips, you are helping to retard the aging process, collagen breakdown, and maintaining more youthful-looking skin while improving your overall health.

Teen Talk...Special Things To Remember

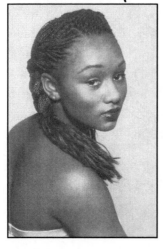

Breaking Out

Pimples and blemishes, blackheads and whiteheads, and discoloration can be problems. If you understand what causes these conditions and know how to cover and remove them effectively and safely, then you will feel better about your face and about yourself.

Other Troublesome Discolorations

Moles

Moles can be removed very easily. Usually when they are removed there is a discoloration that is left for a period of time. Mole removal is not recommended for teens (or adults) who have had keloids in the past. In terms of large scars, if they are keloids, and raised, sometimes repeated injections of cortisone can soften and flatten them, although not remove them completely.

Birthmarks

Birthmarks can be concealed with makeup or treated with lasers, and sometimes surgically removed, but some type of scar probably will remain.

All About Acne

(excerpted from *Natural Radiance: A Guide for Ethnic Skin Care by Pamela Springer*)

Acne is a very commonly occurring skin disease that is characterized by bumps, blackheads and whiteheads, large nodules and cysts.

There are three primary causes of acne: clogging of the pores, overgrowth of a special bacteria that lives on the skin, or overproduction of oil by oil glands or sebaceous glands.

Acne Types

There are only two types of acne – non-inflammatory and inflammatory.

- o Non-inflammatory are lesions that are either blackheads, plugged pores filled with black debris, or whiteheads. Whiteheads may be present as a firm whitish bump on the skin. The material inside this lesion is trapped oil.

- o Inflammatory lesions usually are present with redness, swelling and possibly filled with pus. These blemishes are more serious and may take 8 to 12 weeks to subside. If subsurface lesions, such as nodules or cysts, are present, seek advice from a dermatologist.

Who Gets Acne and the Cause?

Approximately 85% of the population, ages 12 to 24, has had some kind of breakout. Acne is increasing in the female population. Factors may include cosmetic and the fluctuation of hormones prior to their monthly cycle.

However, there may be a number of factors that could attribute to acne lesions.

- o Heredity
- o Increased oil production
- o Bacteria
- o Hormones
- o Build up of dead cells in the pores

Psychological and Social Impact

It is increasingly frustrating to have not only acne but also the residual dark spots. Studies show that there are significant psychological and social impacts on individuals with acne. They tend to be socially withdrawn, lack self-confidence, and have a poor body image. Because of facial lesions, individuals often become embarrassed and withdrawn. Statistics reveal a higher rate of unemployment amongst teens that are presented with acne.

Remedies:
Get on a good acne regimen using products that contain zinc, sulfur, and salicylic.

The mainstay of therapy revolves around Benzoyl Peroxide products, which come in the form of cleansers, gels and lotions, ranging in concentration from the low end of 2.5 percent to the high end of 10 percent. The lower concentration is most often recommended, unless your skin is extremely oily. *Be careful not to overuse Benzoyl Peroxide. It is known to dry out the skin causing the oil gland to become over-productive due to the lack of water on the skin. This over-production of oil may cause clogging of pores and initiate breakouts.*

There are a variety of both over-the-counter, as well as prescription treatments. Another common over-the-counter product is salicylic acid, which comes in a 2 percent concentration and is tolerated by most skin types.

Prescription acne medications consist of oral antibiotics and topical antibiotics, as well as retinoids, which unclog pores.

Special Stuff:
Have you heard of the triple-oxygen facial? Though quite expensive, it's for all skin types, but it is particularly for acne-prone skin. The oxygen kills surface bacteria to help control breakouts and increase circulation for a healthy glow.

It Gets Worse Before it Gets Better

If you have neglected your skin – particularly if you have oily skin with subliminal blemishes, blackheads, and whiteheads – your complexion may appear to get worse once you begin taking care of it. You may even find pimples you didn't see before. Don't worry. Your skin is a means by which your body rids itself of impurities. So when you cleanse and improve your system, you may well find your body expelling impurities through your facial pores, and this can result in temporary facial skin problems. Also, what you see on your face may be merely the blemishes becoming more visible as the dead outermost layer is removed. Thus, the blemishes are now closer to the surface and more visible – but also easier to address.

Ask Mercedes Fleetwood:

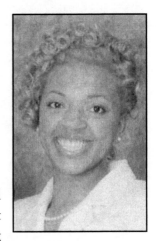

So many people are into temporary and permanent hair removal based on what is portrayed in the media. What is the relationship between hair and skin and what is the difference between all of the different removal systems?

Hair acts as a lubricant in the armpit and pubic region between areas of skin that would otherwise rub together, making life quite uncomfortable for us all. It regulates our internal body temperature by swelling up and making itself thicker while 'clogging' up the pores to hold heat in during the cold weather months and it catches the sweat that is excreted by our pores when our body overheats. This sweat scent is produced in these two areas more than anywhere else in the human body and conveys olfactory information about the producer, which makes them highly, or not-so, attractive to others.

Numerous methods of hair removal fall under two categories: either temporary or permanent. Temporary methods can usually be done in the privacy of your own home and include shaving, trimming, depilatories that chemically dissolve hair, friction, tweezing, waxing, sugaring, threading, or rotary epilators. Permanent methods, which are far more costly, and should only be done by trained, certified professionals, include: electrolysis, laser, flashlamp, and prescription medications. Extensive research into these methods will help you determine which hair removal system is the right choice for you.

How do you get rid of and prevent hair bumps in the bikini area?

Bikini bumps are the result of a few situations: one is ingrown hairs – they pop up when a hair attempts to grow back and push through the outer layer of skin, but instead, gets caught underneath the outer layer of skin and grows curled back into the skin instead of out through the pore. The other two causes are irritation from friction or scabs as a result of the hair removal process of your choice.

To get rid of bikini bumps, you should first discontinue the hair removal method that caused the bumps in the first place. Then you can exfoliate the skin to remove any dead skin cells and encourage the hairs under the skin to grow through the pores. There are numerous products on the market that claim to remove bikini bumps. I would steer clear of any that have alcohol and other harsh chemicals in them since this area is already naturally sensitive and is now irritated from one process.

Common methods (that actually work!) for preventing bikini bumps include soaking the skin in warm water prior to your preferred hair removal process. This will open the pores and lubricate the skin to lessen the possibility of chaffing. If you shave, you should always use a new razor each time and use products specifically formulated for sensitive skin. Also, shave in a downward motion (with the grain) rather than an upward motion (against the grain). This will lessen your chances of experiencing bikini bumps.

Chapter 5

Coloring Your Skin

The most notable differences among people are their size, features, and color. More often than not, we find the widest variation in size, and so generally we don't classify people by size except to say that they're tall or short, fat or thin. However, we do classify people—rightly or wrongly —by their color and features. Those who are dark-skinned and who have negroid features are perceived to be black whether they are or not. Those who have fair or light skin and aquiline features are more often perceived to be white. These shorthand classifications in many ways are useful, but when you apply them to individuals, they have very little value. When you think in terms of make-up, however, they have value, and that is what this chapter is all about.

Your Facial Skin Color

Melanin is the dark pigment in your epidermis, hair, and eyes that help determine your facial, hair, and eye colors. Melanin and your features determine the colors you should wear. For instance, there are critical differences in applying make-up color to your face. If you are African-American, you must consider all three colors, none of which is neutral. You must look at your hair, eyes, and skin color in determining your make-up color.

Let's start at the beginning. Skin color is determined by three factors: carotene, melanin, and hemoglobin. Carotene gives a yellowish tinge to the skin, while melanin lends a brown color and hemoglobin contributes a reddish hue to the skin. The more melanin, the darker the surface skin tone; carotene, on the other hand, provides contrast with a yellow undertone. The tone and undertone to your skin is based on the amount of carotene and melanin in the epidermis. For example, there are Africans from the Sudan who are so dark that they appear to have a bluish aura to their skin. This is directly related to the amount of epidermal melanin and hemoglobin.

All make-up is created to complement the undertone as well as the surface tone of your face. You may have forgotten the basic color chart, but now you need to know that, in terms of primary colors, brown is really a red. There is a range of colors, or shades, that you should use in your make-up, based on the amount and quality of color in your skin. Although the range of possible colors is wide, it is not limitless. Some colors do not go well with other colors. And the more facial colors you have to work with, the more limited your make-up options. The colors you put on your face should go well with the colors of your hair, eyes, and skin and should appeal to your sense of self as well as be appropriate for the occasion.

Skin Color Classifications

Skin color bears a relationship to your natural hair color; therefore, I refer to your natural hair, eye, and skin colors in my analysis. Among women of color are those who are fair-skinned, with blonde or ash-blond to light-brown hair. Then there are women who have medium-light to dark-brown hair. There are also women with dark-brown to black hair. And finally, there are women with blue-black hair. For example, Trinidadians often have "coal black" hair, which has a bluish cast.

The other feature you need to remember in color coding is your eyes. For people of color, the eye range is from green to hazel, blue to hazel, hazel to light brown, dark brown, and very dark brown. Also, people from the Caribbean and sometimes Africa have hazel eyes with a bluish outer rim.

Three Guides, Plus

So far, I have noted the three guides you have in determining what colors to put on your face: your skin tone, your eye color, and your hair color. Those three do not clash with one another. One way or another, they are in harmony, and that is the key. The color you put on your face must harmonize with each feature individually and all three collectively. When this occurs, the invisible fourth guide—the "plus"—comes into play: how you feel and wish to feel.

The Color ABCs

Don' let the myriad of eye shadows, blushers, lipsticks, and nail polishes throw you. There are hundreds of hues but only three basic colors: red, yellow, and blue. This is as important to remember as the fact that black skin generally has one of the following three undertones: yellow, brown, or red-blue, with all their gradations.

You also need to remember that a color will draw from itself. For example, yellow will draw from orange, making the orange look more red. Why does this occur? Since orange is a combination of yellow and red, the yellows are pulled to each other (the yellow in your skin's undertone and the yellow in the color), in a sense leaving the red to stand alone, complementing the yellow.

So, if you have a sallow complexion or a yellow, yellow-red, yellow-beige, or even olive undertone, then red is an inviting color. On the other hand, if you have more of a ruddy complexion, with a more red than yellow undertone, the red draws from the orange, leaving a yellow look. In the same way, if you use green eye shadow and have blue eyes, your eye color drains the blue from the green, leaving a yellow look.

Some colors make you feel warm, vibrant, and alive, while others make you feel cool, "laid back," and somber. There are sufficient colors in each skin, hair, and eye category to permit you to choose the right color for the mood you want.

Certain colors may be more appropriate than others for a particular time of day, occasion, and fashion. You can make the color choices from your category, since each has enough colors from which to select.

Forget the Colors Seasons

You may be surprised that I have not presented colors in terms of seasons of the year. This is because I believe a woman doesn't need a certain season to wear a given color. She can make herself feel like any season she wants. There is no reason why you can't wear "summer" colors in the winter or "spring" colors in the fall. In fact, you will find any color in nature during any season, someplace in the world.

Likewise, don't get caught by the animal stereotype that colors should be more subdued in the winter and brighter in the summer. This camouflage may help animals protect themselves from predators by allowing them to blend into their surroundings. But you are a proud, lovely woman who wishes to make a harmonious statement, so make the statement.

Foundations For Your Skin Type

Like many people, you may think of foundation as concealer. But really it's used to impart a hint of color to your skin. Foundation is sometimes referred to as "base," "base color," or "make-up base."

When I talk to women of color about foundation, I stress that foundation can be used to:

1. Protect against bacteria and impurities.
2. Even out the skin tones—that is, a light T-zone or dark patchy areas.
3. Improve skin texture for a flawless, smooth finish; blushers and other make-up glide on easier and cling better when the skin is covered with a foundation.
4. Kill or decrease sallow skin (a greenish-yellowish or ashy cast), which happens with certain skin pigment types.
5. Create a natural-looking healthy skin glow.

Types of Foundations

Skin Type	Formula	Coverage	Texture
❏ Oily (use oil free base)	Liquid/summer Cream/winter Cream to powder/ summer	Light Medium/total Medium	Matte Semi-matte Matte
❏ Dry (use oil-based make-up)	Pancake cream Soufflé cream Stick/tube Liquid	Total Medium/total Total Sheer/medium	Dewy Dewy Dewy Semi-matte
❏ Combination (use water-based make-up)	Liquid Cream to powder Pancake cream	Sheer Medium/total Total	Semi-matte Matte Dewy
❏ Sensitive (use oil-free, fragrance-free tested make-up)	Liquid Cream to powder	Light Medium	Moist Matte

Make-up Finish

Skin, that looks oily and greasy is not attractive when color is applied. Likewise, dry skin can look dull, sallow, and ashen and will lack a healthy luster without a moist finish. If your skin is very oily and you prefer a finish with no shine or sheen, request a matte make-up finish. If you have normal to combination skin, you may desire an ultra-smooth semi-matte finish (a slight shine). If your skin is dry, strive for a moist dewy finish that will give your skin a natural glow.

During the *extreme hot and humid months* (July and August) in most cities, use these alternatives for relief from very oily skin:

❏ **Clear skin**—light, oil-free moisturizing lotion, with an oil-absorbent, shaded powder.

❏ **Problem skin**—skip the moisturizing step and apply an oil-free liquid foundation, since the oil from your skin is usually sufficient. Use a deep-pore cleanser and deep-pore cleansing mask frequently, with fragrance-free, dermatology-tested powder shades.

Create Your Specific Foundation Look

When you go to a cosmetics counter, especially one in an upscale department store, it is important to inform the beauty advisor or make-up artist what you are looking for and what you can expect from your foundation make-up. There are some specific products that can give you a natural or soft velvet look, or can give coverage to problem skin that will still give you a soft, natural look.

Create a Bare Healthy Glow Look

Bare healthy glow is a foundation finish that is sheer, light in texture, and provides a natural look. If you have normal to combination skin, then a sheer foundation is usually best. You have nothing to hide and have a natural, even-tone skin.

Create a Velvet Glow Look

Light to medium coverage is the foundation coverage for the woman with an uneven skin tone, with blemishes, or with dull patchy areas and visible pores. When you use velvet glow coverage, the skin takes on a very soft, velvet texture.

Create a Smooth Refined Look

This coverage is perfect when your skin has real problems: stretch marks, dark and light spots, superficial scars, dull sallow places, gray patchy areas, and blemishes. When applied properly, this foundation effect can appear very natural, without a masklike, heavy ashen look. (For best results, consult the facial chart in Chapter 2 for movement directions.)

I do not recommend color washes, bronzing gels, or tints and color adjusters for women of color. To date, not enough research has been done on dark skin tones to convince me that these items are beneficial.

Your Skin May Need A Concealer

Facial hair is but one skin condition that many women want to alter. Other features you may find disturbing, if not unsightly, are age spots, blemishes, stretch marks, tattoos, birthmarks, varicose veins, and the like.

Before reading the following material and sections you should go back to Chapter I and read the material on nutrition and your skin. But remember that through good nutrition you can improve the health of your skin and thereby erase, retard, or stop some of these detractions. When this is not possible, or in the interim period during improvement, then you can use cosmetic coverings or concealments. But believe me, you can best improve the condition and look of your skin through diet.

"Normal Skin"

What you might call "perfect" skin, we in the cosmetics field call "normal" skin. Normal skin is facial tissue with few blemishes, and very little roughness or peeling. Many of you may have such skin. Normal skin has a uniform coloration that permits the upper skin layer to admit and reflect light (translucency), with unclogged pores. Some individuals maintain their normal skin all their lives with limited effort. But generally they are the exception. For most people, "normal" skin must be achieved—and it is achievable.

Surface Skin is the Key

It will appear that I am repeating myself, and to some degree I am, but surface skin is the key to a fine appearance. And caring for surface skin can improve it. Clearing the surface of dead cells will improve your skin; under normal conditions, it will perfect the condition of your skin.

Clearing should be done with a mild toner. It actually removes the dead skin, which often is not visible to the eye but gives a look of slight roughness and aging. In contrast, when I mention exfoliating, I refer to an astringent, which some women may need.

It Gets Worse Before It Gets Better

If you have neglected your skin—particularly if you have oily skin with subliminal blemishes, blackheads, and whiteheads—your complexion may appear to get worse once you begin taking care of it. You may even find pimples you didn't see before. Don't worry. Your skin is a means by which your body rids itself of impurities. So when you cleanse and improve your system, you may well find your body expelling impurities through its facial pores, and this can result in temporary facial skin problems. Also, what you see on your face may be merely the blemishes becoming more visible as the dead outermost layer is removed. Thus, the blemishes are now closer to the surface and more visible—but also easier to address.

Using a Concealer

If you are working to clear your skin, you'll see progress eventually, but you may want to use a concealer in the meantime. Let's discuss cover sticks (semiconcealers) and concealers in the pages that follow.

Cover Sticks

A cover stick generally comes as a squeezable tube or lipstick-type tube. In either case, you apply the cream to the spot or area you wish to conceal. The cover stick is generally for mild pigmentations and discolorations.

Cover sticks are excellent tools borrowed from the theater to spot-conceal flaws anywhere on you face, with special consideration for shadows under the eyes, lines around the eyes near the temple, dark eyelids, lines around the nose and mouth, and the cleft in the chin. Cover sticks usually come in beige-yellow tints in light, medium, and dark and are especially blended for women of color. If you have a medium-dark skin tone, use a cover stick a shade darker so as not to play up the often lined and puffy tissue. The goal is to give the illusion that where the dark skin, upper lid, and area under the eyes come together, the skin tone is lighter, softer, and therefore, smoother than it really is. In most cases, I prefer to apply the cover stick on top of foundation. The creams blend better and the cover stick formula stays put longer because it has something to cling to; also, it won't crease, slip around, or bleed. Use your ring finger to gently pat on the cover stick formula, as illustrated on page **. On dry eyelids, use a cover stick to achieve a smoother finish to your eye shadow and to keep the shadow in place. You can also use a cover stick to contour your nose; see the illustration on page **.

Concealers

Many women of color are plagued with scars, pigment discolorations, varicose veins, stretch marks, and the like. The cosmetics industry has discovered this and has done an outstanding job in providing quality products for women with these conditions. Concealers are waterproof coverups for large areas.

Iman, Flori Roberts and Fashion Fair Cosmetics, respectively, have revolutionized the cosmetics industry with their concealing products keyed to the dark pigmentation of African-Caribbean, African-Latin, African-European, and African-American women—a real breakthrough. Flori Roberts' Derma Blend is especially formulated to cover leg veins and stretch marks. Fashion Fair introduced concealing cream shades called Cover Tone that blend easily with shades in their liquid, cream, and pancake cream foundations. For all skin types, these corrective creams are waterproof, non-greasy, and smudge-free (a plus for oily skin). They easily conceal most skin imperfections, such as scars, burn marks, blotches, blemishes, undereye shadows, age spots, birthmarks, broken capillaries, varicose veins, stretch marks, surgical discolorations, and tattoos.

I will now suggest how to apply a concealer for maximum effect. First, you skin has to be "squeaky clean." The manufacturers supply directions for their products, but they all say basically the same thing: clean skin is a must before application; apply concealer directly to the affected area using a spatula that generally comes with the product; apply the product a little at a time.

If you don't like to use the spatula, use your hands to apply the concealer, but make absolutely sure that both hands are clean. Apply the product with your fingertips and gently spread a light covering over the entire area so that the treated area is indistinguishable in color from the surrounding skin. You may find that by warming the product in your hands (the palm), it can be applied easier. Always start at the center of the area and move outward. When the concealer completely covers the area, and is properly matched, it will almost melt and blend into your natural color.

While the concealer is still damp, immediately apply the specially formulated powder in order to set, seal, and dry the concealer. All of this must be done before you can touch the area. It shouldn't take more than a minute to apply the concealer and powder. As long as the concealer is applied rapidly and is still damp when you begin with the powder, you are safe.

Now you can decide whether you wish to use a foundation. Most women will. Apply your foundation along the outer edge of the concealed area. Blend it in there and over the rest of your face.

The key to successful use of a concealer is to pair the right concealer and foundation with your skin color. Then you can blend at the edges, or demarcation line, to achieve a flawless look.

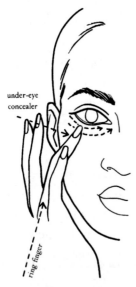

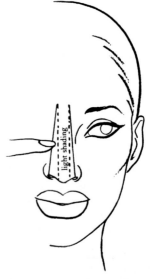

Use your ring finger to apply under-eye concealer or cover stick beneath the eye or above the eyelid, moving left to right. The cover stick can also serve as a foundation for eye shadow.

Apply light cover stick down the center of your nose. Apply darker cover stick or contour powder on each side of your nose, shading the nostril area. Gently blend with your fingertip and set with powder.

Blending Your Foundation

This is a very important step. When I say "blending," that is exactly what I mean: placing the color next to your skin and having it look natural. For example, many women mistakenly apply foundation first to their chin. Instead, they should apply less foundation to the chin so that there is closer harmony with the skin on the neck. You should always blend your foundation downward, with less and less foundation at the chin area. Always blend downward and blend lightly. The downward movement allows for better coverage because of the way facial hairs lie on the skin and hair without streaking.

If you are using a liquid foundation, place four dots of it on your face, then blend them together. (If you have oily skin, and are using an oil-free product, be aware that you must use it rapidly because these products dry quickly—in approximately 30 seconds. If you are too slow, the dots will dry and you will be able to see where you placed them on your face.) The four-dot method is the best approach because you will not use too much foundation, and you will develop a rapid way of getting complete and natural coverage on your face. One mistake many women of color make is to put on too much foundation, believing this is the only way to get total coverage. Instead, put one dot on the forehead, one on each cheek, and one on the chin; maybe add one on the tip of the nose (this would be a fifth dot). Use your fingertips and blend the dots into each other, working out to the hairline and jawline.

The best tool for applying a soufflé, cream, or pancake cream foundation is a sponge. I am a firm believer in using a sponge. It is clean and it frees the hands; it is better than your fingertips because the warmth of your fingers can cause streaking. But don't wipe your skin with the sponge. Use a press, dab, and pat movement (see the following illustration). This allows you to place the proper amount of color where it's needed.

As you know, a sponge has holes, and as you press the sponge onto the surface of the foundation, it lifts away the product. So press quickly, lift quickly, and apply to the face. I don't recommend sponges for applying a liquid foundation, though, because they have a tendency to absorb too much liquid. Once you apply the liquid foundation with your fingertips, however, you can go back over your work with a damp sponge to smooth your foundation to the finish you want.

For those women who use a soufflé with a liquid cream, a cream, or the pancake foundation, the sponge is the best tool for application. The cream stick is another item that can be applied to your face with a sponge.

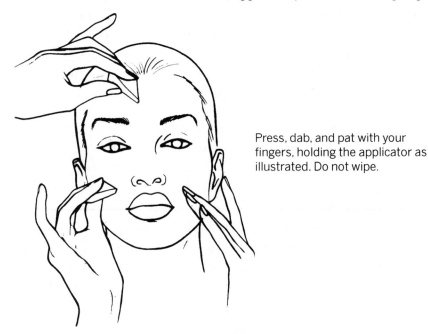

Press, dab, and pat with your fingers, holding the applicator as illustrated. Do not wipe.

If you are like many women, you probably use a thick, round sponge that's sold at most cosmetic counters. And if you are like the many women who have spoken to me, you probably find these sponges cumbersome. You have to fold them in half and press them to your skin. Sometimes they unfold, slip, crumble, and even come apart. Why use a big sponge when you use only half—and that half with difficulty? Besides, the round sponge is very difficult to clean. There are square sponges, but most women find them too flat and, again, too cumbersome. The ideal sponge is triangular, so that it can be held between the index and middle finger and the thumb. Use a triangular sponge, employing the technique of press, dab, and pat. Don't wipe, scrub, or use a rubbing motion.

Placing the Foundation on Your Face

Where and how you place the foundation is very important. Once again, think in terms of facial zones. The center zone of your face is called the T-zone, and it is here that you should start to apply the foundation. Begin at the forehead and move toward the temples and around the eye area.

Circle around the eye area as if to get an owl-eye look. You don't want to put foundation on the eyelids or under the eye—just up to the rim of this area. The reason for using this owl-eye approach is that ingredients in some formulations might affect such sensitive areas.

If you have blemishes in these areas, use a cover stick or a concealer as a foundation for eye shadow and to erase any darkness under the eyes. Remember: your application movements should always be outward toward the hairline, but the stroking, pressing, dabbing, and patting motions are lightly downward. This will encourage any facial hair to lie flat, since hair usually grows downward. Movement then is from the center of the T-zone, blending the forehead, temples, and under the eyes, then moving to the cheeks and then lightly from the cheekbone down toward the jawline.

You should lighten your application when reaching the jawline, so that your foundation blends evenly below the jaw. There should be no demarcation line between the jawline and the neck. You do not—and should not—carry the foundation beneath the chin and jawline onto the throat and neck. I repeat: application is from the center of your face outward toward the hairline. The movements are press, dab, and pat, stroking lightly downward to press the hair down.

The Neck Area

For over twenty-five years I have been against putting foundation on the neck; I am still against it, because there is no reason to do it. When the cosmetic chemist keys color to your facial area, he or she uses the color tones in the center of your face, and moves outward toward the hairline to determine your undertone. Skin colors vary greatly in terms of shading at the temples, at the center of the face, on the jawline, and on the neck. You can't judge facial color based on the color of your hands, arms, neck or jaw—they are generally all different. So if you want a true facial color tone, you must go by the suggestions I make for matching skin color to proper foundation.

There are but a few exceptions to what I have just stated. If you have an extremely light face, which is much lighter than your neck, then select a foundation that is a little darker, so as to match the dark tones of your neck. If your face is darker and neck lighter, then you should choose a foundation just a little lighter. It may look a little strange at the center of your face when you apply it initially, but as you blend the foundation in, you will see how it complements the neck color.

With this method, your facial color, foundation, and neck color will blend. Remember: when someone looks at you, he or she doesn't stare at your face or neck unless you do something striking to draw the person's eye. What people do, however, is look at you in a general way. You may recall I said at the beginning of this chapter that people look at each other and classify one another. They look for impressions. If you make the areas close to the temples and jawline blend with the neck color, whether darker or lighter than your face, you will convey the impression that both are the same color. It is the eyes' impression that you are after.

Another reason why you should not color your neck is that the cosmetics will soil your clothing. I have found this to be a serious problem for so many women who apply foundation or powder to their necks.

Option: For severe neck discoloration, the smudge-proof/water-proof color coded concealers are alternatives.

How To Choose Your Foundation

Women of color should choose a foundation that perfectly matches their skin tone. To be able to choose properly, first there are some "don'ts" you should avoid.

❑ Don't try to change your skin tone with foundation. Models, actresses, entertainers, and opera stars often have to change their skin tone for stage effect. However, most women appear in natural light or artificial light. It is important to choose a foundation that coordinates and harmonizes with your skin tone.

❏ Don't buy a foundation without testing several colors in you skin-tone range. Test them in natural and artificial light.

❏ Don't buy one foundation and expect it to impart the right color for four seasons of the year.

❏ Don't wear your friends' foundations. If a friend is in your color range, she might have yellow-olive undertones whereas you might have yellow-red. The foundation will be different, therefore.

❏ Don't rush your purchase. You can't rush into a store on the tail end of your lunch hour and quickly choose the foundation, especially if it's your first time or you have developed new color problems. You must take the time and have the patience to test your foundation, but first check your skin for changes and buy foundation accordingly.

Now that those don'ts are out of the way, here's what you should do.

First, because your skin is dark, it is important that you test a foundation based on the season in which it is to be worn. As your skin gets darker or lighter it can take on a golden-red, reddish brown, or brownish blue undertone based on the amount of sun or wind it is exposed to. Don't look for an exact match; you are not involved in true skin-tone match-ing. For example, in the summer I suggest a summer foundation that cools down the yellow, red, and blue undertones.

Your true skin tone can be tested for accuracy during the latter part of the fall and in the winter months. The situation is different, however, for light, medium, and dark skin tones, for they turn sallow, olive-brown, or deepish yellow-gray or brown. I suggest a winter foundation that imparts golden-beige, copper-brown, and rich red-brown radiance to dark skin tones.

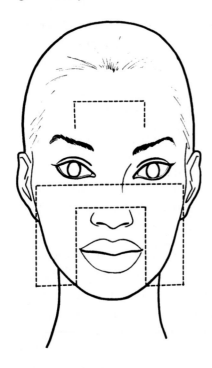

Test the center of your face, cheeks, and jawline to determine a perfect foundation match.

Second, you should be aware that there are numerous cosmetics companies marketing skin-bleaching agents to women of color. These products permit you to even out your skin tone or fade out blotches and superficial spots. The bleaching product blends the shades of the spot and the surrounding skin. These creams also lighten the outer layer, giving an appearance of lighter skin.

When you use these bleaching creams, there is something to remember. Your skin takes on a more yellowish undertone, since you have bleached out the dark part of the brown pigment in the melanin. This slight difference means you must rematch your foundation.

Third, you should know the effects of your medications. Birth-control pills will darken large parts of your face. Medicine for high blood pressure will sometimes cause the skin to take on a deeper, reddish brown or gray-brown undertone. A liver condition, excessive alcohol consumption, and drug abuse will darken a large section of your face. When such conditions take place, you must revise your foundation. You may have to change the shade until your skin color returns to normal.

Last, make an appointment with a make-up artist or beauty advisor in a retail store or salon. Have the individual do a full-scale make-up application.

Your skin's undertone, as discussed earlier, is the aura or glow of your true skin tone. It can be flushed out by standing in a room or in front of a white wall, with white background, and in natural light. Wrap your hair with your whitest scarf or drape your neck and shoulders with a white sheet. Allow the ultraviolet light to bounce on your face until you can actually see a green (olive), yellow, reddish yellow, reddish brown, or blue aura.

Your Skin Tone and its Undertone

❑ **Light skin**. Fair—undertones yellow and olive; light skin—undertones yellow, red, and ruddy.

❑ **Medium skin**. Light or medium skin—undertones yellow-sallow; medium skin—undertones yellow to red and ruddy.

❑ **Dark skin**. Medium dark skin—undertones golden, brown, and gray; deep dark skin—undertones red, brown, and blue.

Face Powders

Many women of color have decided that they do not need or cannot use powder, largely because they have gotten poor results. However, powder can eliminate the shine for those women whose skin tends to be slightly oily.

Applying powder to your foundation also prepares your face, giving it a silky texture on top of which to apply your blush. However, some make-up artists want you to apply foundation first, other colors next, and powder last, to set the face.

Which method you use depends on your skin type. Those with oily skin should apply powder immediately after the foundation; those with dry skin should apply the foundation first, then the eye and cheek color, and set the face with translucent powder.

Types of Powder

There are two types of powder, and they have different purposes beyond that of setting your foundation: translucent setting powders and shaded, or pigmented, powders. Translucent powders are usually loose formulas, with a tint of either amber or bronze. These are usually termed translucent because you can see through the powder to your skin, which will have a glow. These setting powders are used to absorb surface oil and perspiration—for example, for touch ups before work, after lunch, on the T-zone, and on the cheeks.

Shaded powders are for women who prefer to use a moisturizer and may not use a liquid, cream, or pancake cream foundation. They may be bought either loose or solid in a compact. Shaded powder is applied over your moisturizer, and is a pigmented powder.

Remember, though, that pigmented powder not keyed to your foundation coloring can disturb it. For instance, if you have a bronze foundation and you put a sable powder over it, the result will be a muddy look, giving a gray, dull appearance to the skin. In contrast, translucent powders need not match your color skin. They are designed to set the foundation and absorb the perspiration and oil deposits associated with the foundation.

In summary, some people want to have moist-looking skin while others want a semi-matte or matte appearance. If you don't want a shine, use powder. The option is yours.

The Benefits of Powder

I have already presented some of the benefits of powder, but now I would like to detail additional ones so that you will know what kind of powder to buy, which brand, and what to avoid. Let's review the already noted benefits of powder:

1. Sets make-up foundation
2. Absorbs oil and perspiration
3. Does away with the shine

In addition, today's powders will not dry your skin. Many women of color feel that powder causes a gray or ashy look. This is not true. Most powders have some type of moisturizing agent, and the amount depends on the brand. When properly applied, powders will impart a natural, translucent sheen to the face.

It is important that women with dark skin use only translucent powder after applying foundation. You don't want to employ shaded powders to dust or set your foundation. Also, remember that a little powder goes a long way. You don't need to use a lot of powder to set your foundation. A "cakey" effect is not attractive, and it emphasizes any lines you have under you eyes, around the nose and mouth, and even the cleft of the chin. Think of putting a sheer veil over your face; that is the amount of powder to apply. The ideal is to use powder to set the foundation, and to allow the skin and color foundation to glow.

How to Apply Powder

Loose powder comes in a container with a scoop-out feature, so it can be reused and so as not to spoil the entire product. A shaker container is ideal for some women; the powder can actually be shaken out of the container. It is like a salt or pepper shaker, whereby you can measure the amount of powder and control its spillage. There is also a compact powder. In this instance, you cannot shake or pour the powder, but rather, you use a flat puff applicator to lift the powder from the container to your face.

A cotton ball is usually used to apply loose or pressed powder. A powder puff is usually flat and is used for applying pressed powder. The fluffy powder puff is usually used for loose powder, while the fluffy powder brush, which is an ideal applicator, is recommended highly for loose or pressed powder application.

How to Get the Look You Want

What look do you want? The matte look is achieved with loose powder and the fluffy puff. Press, dab, and pat is again the operation in applying loose powder (see illustration on page **). To achieve a sheen (a moist look), again use loose powder but apply with a powder brush. To achieve an oil-free, perspiration-free look, women with oily skin, or women who do not want a shine in the T-zone, use pressed powder with a flat puff or a cotton ball. Pressed powder, in general, is ideal for oil absorption; in fact, there are pressed powders designed for oil absorption. You should ask for these particular formulas at your cosmetics counter if you are trying to rid your skin of perspiration and oil.

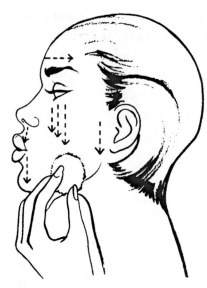

Use a powder puff to press, dab, and pat your face with powder, using downward strokes to encourage any fine hairs to lie smooth and even.

Once again, let's make sure you understand that there should be no scrubbing, no rubbing. To do this only takes off your make-up and redeposits it, usually in the very places you don't want it.

Some Powder Tricks

Use a loose powder whenever you want to take away a line of demarcation. These are usually under the eyes, along the hairline, and on the jawline. Loose powder is excellent for blending your under-eye concealer with your blusher. Setting powder can easily be powdered between these two lines to soften the effect, or even erase it, to become a very natural meeting of color. The trick is to dip the powder brush in the powder and flick away the excess powder, then redip the brush in the loose powder and flip away the loose powder, and then dip the brush into the blusher and shake off the excess. Now you have both the blusher color and the loose powder on the bristles. All you have to do is fan the brush over the line of the demarcation and get a softened effect.

Teen Talk...
Special Things To Remember

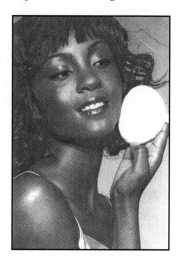

Love Your Facial Skin Color

Now that you understand what a good skincare regimen consists of, it's time for the "411" on achieving your most stunning look. Your skin color or tone is the key.

Makeup is created to complement the undertone as well as the surface tone of your face...but you must choose carefully. Teens today can change their hair color and can appear to have changed their eye color by wearing tinted contact lenses; but your natural beauty starts with your natural tone and undertone. The right foundation will help you enhance that beauty.

Create Your Specific Foundation Look

When you go to the cosmetics counter, especially one in an upscale department store, it is important to inform the beauty adviser or makeup artist of what you are looking for and what you expect from your foundation. If your skin is very oily and you prefer a finish with no shine or sheen, request a matte makeup finish. If you have normal-to-combination skin, you may desire an ultrasmooth semi-matte finish (a slight shine). If your skin is dry, ask for a moist, dewy finish that will give your skin a natural velvet glow.

One mistake many teens make is to use too much foundation, believing this is the only way to get total coverage. If you are using a liquid foundation, place five dots on your face, then blend them together. Put one dot on the forehead, one on each cheek, one on the chin, and one on the tip of the nose. Use your fingertips and blend the dots into one another, working out to the hairline and jawline.

Ordinarily, you should not have to put foundation on your neck. Your facial color, foundation and neck color will blend unless you have severe discoloration.

The best tool for applying a soufflé, cream, pancake cream foundation or a cream stick is a sponge. Use a press, dab and pat movement; don't wipe, scrub or use a rubbing motion. The ideal sponge is triangular so that it can be held between the index finger and thumb.

The Benefits of Powder

1. Sets makeup foundation
2. Absorbs oil and perspiration
3. Does away with the shine
4. Blushers glide on more easily and set better

Face Powder

Remember that a little powder goes a long way. You don't need to use a lot of powder to set your foundation. A "cakey" effect is not attractive, and it emphasizes any lines you have under your eyes, around the nose and mouth, and even the cleft of your chin.

A fluffy powder brush is an ideal applicator for both the loose and pressed (compact) powders.

QUIZ

Q. *What is the primary reason to use foundation?*
A. To even out your skin tone.

Q. *What are the three most important steps to your daily regimen?*
A. Cleanse, tone and moisturize

Q. *What does translucent powder do?*
A. Sets your makeup and gives you a matte finish

Q. *What is the best way to tone down blemishes or dark marks?*
A. Apply concealer after you moisturize your skin.

Q. *What should I drink to help keep my skin clear?*
A. Eight glasses of water a day

Ask Mercedes Fleetwood:

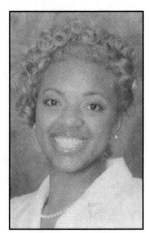

My skin is very blotchy. I am looking for a foundation that will give me the most coverage, yet look natural. What do you suggest?

Many women of color have uneven skin tones and blotchiness. With so many great products on the market, most of these conditions can be easily concealed with a foundation. If the discoloration is too much to cover with foundation alone, blend on a cover stick or concealer first. I find that the mousse or crème to powder makeups give great coverage, but many of my friends are now using bare minerals and they love it. The main consideration is finding the color that works for your complexion. Always try it before you buy it. Natural is the look you want to achieve; you should never look like you are wearing a mask.

Chapter 6

Coloring Your Face

Now that you have applied your foundation, you are ready to do your eyes, cheeks, and lips. But in order to color your face, you need the proper tools.

Your Color Tools

The tools that I discuss here may, in some instances, be different from those you have previously used. However, these are the ones I believe are the easiest and most functional.

- o Powder brush
- o Eye shadow brush
- o Blush brush
- o Brow brush
- o Contour brush

- o Lash comb
- o Eyeliner brush
- o Lip liner pencil
- o Eye shadow sponge
- o Lipstick brush

The right equipment is important, but you also must know the proper techniques and procedures. Your make-up steps now come into full use. In the previous chapters we discussed skin care, foundations, and powders. Now is the time you begin to apply what you have learned. I know that many of you will have your own techniques and procedures already, but I urge you to compare your methods with what I am about to propose. And for those of you who have no method, or who have been confused by the myriad of products put in front of you, I offer the following steps:

1. Cleanse
2. Tone
3. Moisturize
4. Apply concealer
5. Apply foundation, or base
6. Contour the cheeks
7. Apply powder

After the above steps, you might want to apply eye make-up. Next, apply blusher and then lipstick. Some women prefer a different order; they might go to the blusher, then to the eyes, and then do the lips. The choice is yours.

Your Eyes and the Use of Color

When I think of eyes, I think of Erykah Badu, Brandy, Vivica Fox, Tyra Banks, Angela Bassett, Vanessa Williams, Rhianna, Alicia Keys, Beyonce, and Halle Berry—all with eyes that allure, that hold, capture, and hypnotize you.

These are the faces of visible African-American women, and their eyes are made up to hold our attention. Because of this, many women tend to admire and sometimes yearn to look like them. I understand this, but I disagree. These beautiful women are made up for the world of films, entertainment, and fashion. They do not live your lifestyle.

Refined, secure women show themselves by making a clear, natural, never overcolored statement to the world. They dress and use color based on the occasion. They are about serious business. They are striving to be the best they can—at work, in their social affairs, at home, and in church. They should achieve notice through the quality of their performance, not through garish make-up or inappropriate use of color. Now, let's begin to dress your eyes with appropriate color.

How to Apply Eye Make-up

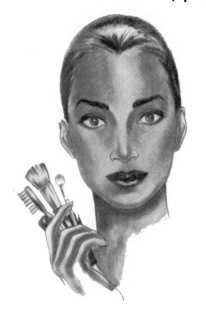

I have designed a simple system for you. It is a four-step, full-scale rainbow eye system in which we consider the correct approach to the eye shape, eyeliner, and lash application. The major principle is to keep the look clean, blended, and subtle. The exception is with evening make-up, when you should exaggerate to shine and sparkle, when *pizzazz* is the operative word. Here is the order for applying eye make-up:

1.   Eyeliner
2.   Eye shadow
3.   Mascara
4.   Eyebrow make-up

Eyeliner

Eyeliners come in formulas designed for each skin type and in different forms: soft pencil, liquid, cream, and pressed cake.

Eyeliners are used to give more definition to the eyes. They highlight the eyes and make the eyelashes appear fuller and thicker. A person can really bring the desired effect to the eyes with a liner; it is the ultimate groomer because it separates the shadow from the lashes via a circle around the eyes.

I think a smoldering and smoky look around the eyes is most attractive on women, especially darker-skinned women. Eyeliners to some degree have been in disfavor because of how they are sometimes worn, giving the eyes a thick and harsh look. But now there are many shades in complementary neutral tones. Rich, deep blues look exceptionally well on women with medium to dark skin tones. When you use the eyeliner, be sure to color the top lid as well as the bottom.

There is a technique I would like to suggest, especially to those of you who have problems finding an eyeliner to complement your various shades of eye shadow or your pupils. Take your eye shadow color—maybe the corresponding shade in a dual kit—and simply wet your brush, then stroke the cake of eye shadow for your eyeliner color. For example, if for evening wear you want to use a reddish eye shadow close to the lash, with a dominant red eyeliner that has a little gold in it, moisten your brush and then stroke with the golden-red eye shadow; draw in the color and, presto, you have an eyeliner in a corresponding shade.

Pencil vs. Liquid Eyeliners

Liquid eyeliner is still one of the most popular forms, but I recommend the pencil eyeliner because you can control it better. Pencils come in more colors, they can be smudged on the top and bottom of the eyelids; and they can be applied either thick or thin. If you have had very little practice applying liquid eyeliner, you can easily lose control. Yet both forms are serviceable and can have attractive results.

Purchasing Your Eyeliner

The eyeliner should be color coordinated with your eye shadow. Eyeliners, especially pencils, can be tested at the cosmetics counter. Testing foundations as well as eye, cheek, and lip colors is permitted in department stores, chain stores, and some pharmacies. And you should test the colors. Try to test them in natural light, even if you have to stroke the color on your face or eyelid and then excuse yourself to walk to where there is natural light. Use your make-up mirror to look at the color on your skin, and you will see that in different lighting the shades appear differently.

Just two words of caution. There are waterproof eyeliners that tend to be a little rubbery, but they are excellent if you perspire heavily, if your skin is oily, or if you go swimming a lot. However, I have found that when used frequently these waterproof eyeliners can actually dry out the area around your eyes, leaving it sensitive. This is especially true for those who suffer from allergies or who are naturally sensitive in this area. If this is your situation, then I suggest you avoid the waterproof eyeliners.

Eye Shadow

Eye shadow comes in cream, crayon, powder, or liquid. The powder shadows are ideal for most skin types because they can be controlled easily and they appear to be softer, silkier, and smoother on your skin. However, the powders are best suited for oily, combination, and normal to oily skin.

The cream shadows are best for women with very dry eyelids. The only caution is that women with medium to dark skin tones stay away from creams that have a silver or white talc base, since these shadows give the eye area an ashen look. The light materials play up the gritty, chafed areas and dry lines of your eyelids.

The crayon shadows are excellent for smoothing on and blending in. They can be very soft, and that is the caution for those of you who have oily skin. Make sure you don't overuse an oil-based crayon shadow, for it can build up a crease and melt on the eyelids.

There are several cosmetics companies that encourage customers to dampen their powder eye shadows because it gives it a different consistency and helps them glide on evenly, dry well, and stay put.

There are fragrance-free eye shadows for those of you who have sensitive eyes or tend to have an allergy-prone eye area.

There are eye shadows that are sold as dual kits: two pans containing two colors that usually are a highlighter and a fashion shade, which can also be used for contours. Then there are four-pan color kits: highlighter, contour, and a fashion shade in a light and a dark hue. You can even find six- and twelve-color pan kits that permit you to mix and blend shades to come up with original colors for a rainbow eye, smoldering eye, or contour eye.

Highlighters do not have to be eggshell white or creamy white. They can be pink or dark lavender, or a light shade of blue or even a dark shade of blue. The highlighter you use depends on the effect you want.

Basic eye color application

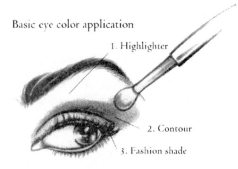

1. Highlighter

2. Contour

3. Fashion shade

A. For a basic eye color effect, apply highlighter, contour, and then fashion shade.

Multicolored eye

1. highlighter

2. Contour

3. Fashion shade

B. For a rainbow, multicolored effect, apply highlighter, contour, and then the fashion eye color.

A. To make your eyes less round:
Liner
Draw a thin line at just the very outer corner of the upper lid and across the bottom lid.
Shadow
Use lots of color, edging shades into the contour crease, shading up and out at the corner.

B. To make eyes more prominent:
Liner
Draw a line from the center of the upper lid out toward the corner. Add a line across the bottom lid.
Shadow
Add a light color to the eyebone, contour color in crease, and use a frosted or light shade on the lid.

C. To make eyes look deeper:
Liner
Draw eyeliner across the top lid and from the center to the outer corner. Apply mascara.
Shadow
Add lots of color in the contour crease. Do not apply light frosted shades.

D. To make small eyes look larger:
Liner
Circle the top and bottom inner lids with soft black, deep blue, or rich deep brown; all three colors will make the white of the eyes appear even whiter and the eyes appear wider. Apply mascara.
Shadow
Color is applied to the eyebone under the brow arch, fanning out toward the temples. Contour color in crease and along the lid as illustrated.

Mascara

The purpose of mascara is to build up your lashes. Mascara makes your lashes look longer, thicker, and more smoldering. There is a formulation that comes as a cream, which I recommend.

The shades that look best on women of color are black, brown/black, dark brown, antique bronze, and berry shades.

Pay attention to your mix of colors when you make up. Be careful what color eye shadow you use with a colored mascara. There should be some coordination of colors between the lashes and the eyelid itself.

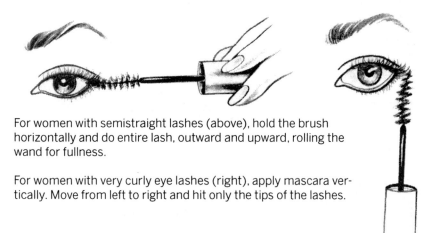

For women with semistraight lashes (above), hold the brush horizontally and do entire lash, outward and upward, rolling the wand for fullness.

For women with very curly eye lashes (right), apply mascara vertically. Move from left to right and hit only the tips of the lashes.

Remember to test the mascara before you buy, but don't allow the beauty adviser to apply it from the tester wand directly to your eyelashes. This tester wand has been used on other women, and any bacteria it picked up from them is in the tube. Bacteria grow extremely fast in the dark warm tubes on the lighted cosmetics counter. That tester wand could put bacteria on your eyes, so make sure you get a clean wand. Cosmetics companies provide disposable wands for testing purposes.

Eyebrow Make-up

Blessed is the woman who does not have gaps and scars in her eyebrows. She does not need make-up. If you are one of these women, then all you have to do is groom and shape your eyebrows with a brush. However, for most women eyebrow make-up fills in the spaces between the hairs and covers any scarring in the brow area.

Eyebrows can easily be filled in with a pencil to give more definition to the line. But don't think in terms of starting at the beginning of your brow and drawing a line to the end, out toward the temples. This is shaping the brow, and in Chapter 4 there is an explanation of how to shape the eyebrow with tweezing. Now you'll just be filling in the spaces between the hair, according to the existing shape. See the following illustration for instructions on filling in sparse eyebrows.

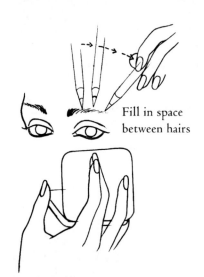

Fill in space between hairs

Eyebrow make-up can also be used where you have overtweezed or overplucked. Shape the eyebrow with the pencil and fill in until new growth appears, then do your reshaping. Also, don't be afraid to experiment with the eyebrow. Some eyebrows look great brushed straight up, toward the hairline; just brush them up and fan them out toward the temples. This is a great look, especially for evening.

For sparse eyebrows, fill in spaces, moving from inner corner of the eyebrow outward.

Blushers

The purpose of a blusher is to bring a blush and glow to the cheeks. I recommend using blushers because they bring a vibrancy and alive quality to your face. But you must carefully select the color and place it correctly.

Don't be dissuaded from using blusher because you see intense color compacts on display at retail cosmetics counters. They are usually very bright or very intense, but you will be surprised how, when keyed to your skin color, those deep, rich pigmented blushers bring a soft natural glow to your cheeks.

Your lipstick and blusher do not have to match; however, they should be of the same color family or in the same color range. For example, a red-brown blusher enhances a yellow-based red lipstick. For evening, a true red blusher with golden highlights makes a wonderful partner to a gold-frosted red lipstick with a golden gloss. With this combination your cheeks and lips will be all aglow with golden sparkle, reflecting light against your dark skin.

Powder Blushers

Powder imparts a natural-looking, soft-matte finish. Of all the formulas, it is the easiest to apply and looks the best on dark skin. Powders glide on smoothly and don't leave a bumpy, ashen buildup. Literally hundreds of powder blushers are available, tailored for every skin type. If you try a blusher that gives a gray appearance to your skin, you can be sure it was not designed for your skin coloring. All skin types can wear powder blusher; however, they are best for those with combination or oily skin. Women with sensitive skin must be very careful, and only use blushers designed for sensitive skin (usually fragrance- and oil-free formulas).

Cream Blushers

There are two basic cream blushers—regular and oil-free—and they come as a swivel stick or in a compact. Use your fingers or the swivel stick for best application. Apply the cream over your foundation and then add your translucent powder. In general, cream blushers are easy to blend, but avoid the pale shades, red to pinks, and peachy to orange colors, because they appear to be suspended in air or to sit on top of the skin.

Cream blushers are best for combination or dry skin. Oily skin collects the shine and high humidity, and in summer months the cheeks appear greasy and slick—not attractive at all! All skin types should stay away from the frosted cream blushers unless the frost is gold, not silver. I don't think silver enhances medium to dark complexions and it should never be used on the cheeks.

Types of Blushers

Type of Blush	Finish	Coverage	Type of Skin	How to Apply
Gel tint	Smooth sheen, gold-frosted gels look great at night; don't ever wear frost during the day	Sheer, light texture; should not be deeply pigmented	Combination to oily (most are oil-free and water-based); not advised for very dry skin; can appear shiny and slick	Use fingertips, on top of foundation, before powder; dry-down period is extremely fast, so you have to work quickly; gel can streak and blotch
Liquid	Moist and smooth	Sheer, light to medium texture; deeply pigmented	All skin types; best suited for combination, medium to dry skin	Use sponge, sliding on top of foundation, then set with powder; easy to apply
Mousse	Soft, dewy-looking; gold-frosted is good at night	Sheer, foam is light textured; not deeply pigmented	Not for dry skin; for oily or combination skin	Use fingertips; blend with a sponge, especially around the edges
Cream	Smooth, dewy; gold-frosted is excellent, some even appropriate for day; best for evening wear, and silver-frosted is out forever!	Medium; deeply pigmented; should not ever appear greasy or slick	Normal to dry skin; oil-free best suited for oily only	Use fingertips and blend on top of foundation, set with powder

Type of Blush	Finish	Coverage	Type of Skin	How to Apply
Powder	Matte or semi-matte frost; gold-frosted is best to highlight cheekbones at night	Medium; deeply pigmented	All skin types; oily skin benefits the most	Use brush; see illustration on page **

Use Blushers with Moderation

Many women wear too much blusher during the day. The ideal application is only a suggestion, or hint, of color. Select rich, pure colors such as copper-bronze with its deep gold base, or a soft plum, light wine-burgundy, or deeply pigmented almond orange shade. When you apply powder blusher, always dip the brush quickly and flick or twist your wrist to stroke the cheek lightly. Remember: it is better to apply just a little blusher and then go back and apply more if you need it, than to apply too much and have to disturb the foundation to remove the excess. Matte colors (no shine) are best for day on all skin types.

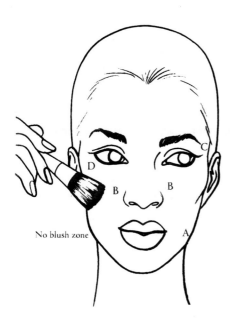

No blush zone

Special Tips:

1. Use the outer corner (A) as a guide to start adding blusher

2. Never apply blusher in the No Blush Zone (B).

3. Always move across, upward, and out toward the hairline (C).

4. Do not add blusher underneath the eyes near the lower rim (D).

Color Placement

The cheek, according to your facial shape and size, is where you should place the blusher. Don't place it on the nose. After all, why put blusher where it will make you look like you have a cold?

The outer corner of your eye is your guideline for application. See the following illustration. Don't ever bring the color toward the broad nostril of your nose; it will ring and broaden your facial structure. Likewise, blusher should not ever be shaded down past the tip of your nose. Draw an imaginary line from the tip of your nose, under your natural cheekbone, to the middle part of your ear; this is usually where you should cut off the shading. Also, most women have a convex eye area, so don't bring the blusher too close to the outer eyes. When applied close to the eyes blushers tend to make them look puffy and drawn.

Square Face:

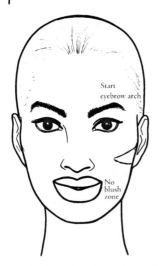

Start eyebrow arch

No blush zone

You have a firm structure, usually a wide forehead, cheeks, and jawline. The apple, or round part of the cheekbone, registers near the outer corner of your eye. Begin the blusher application at this point, sweeping the cheek color wide upward to the center part of the ear.

To soften a wide and square face, apply cheek color at the bottom side of the jaw, with the cheekbone to accent the center of your face. Don't ever apply blusher between the No Blush Zone apple of the cheekbone and the bloom of the nostril.

Your eyebrows are most important. No straight thin lines. Arch your brows at the outer corner of the pupil, looking straight into the mirror, so they are in line with your cheekbones.

Round Face:

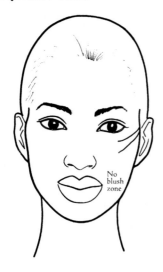

You have a solid structured face. Keep color high on the cheekbone, sweeping it outward and upward to the top of the ear and hairline. Don't ever place color on the apple and never bring color from the apple toward the bloom of the nostril.

You want to discourage a clownish appearance. Keep color high on the top side of the cheekbone. Sweep blusher from the outer corner of the eye, fanning upward. Eyebrows should be naturally full and shaped horizontally with a slight curve. The rainbow eye placed diagonally plays down circles. Shading is appropriate at the temples. The eyes are the facial point: keep lip pencil line faint and inside the natural lip line.

Oval Face:

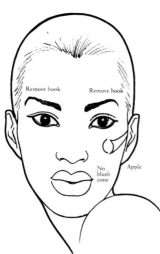

You have the so-called balanced facial structure. Polish the cheekbone with rich, radiant color, sweeping from the outer edge of the corner of your eye and cresting for a V effect. The open part of the V spreads wide toward the ear and hairline.

Play up the apple, moving straight across and fanning outward. Eyebrows take on a subtle half-moon shape. Accentuate the crease and create a more concave illusion. Highlight with greasy mascara. Place shading color at the temples, on tip of the nose, and at chin. Lips are shaped, moist, and dewy.

Narrow Face:

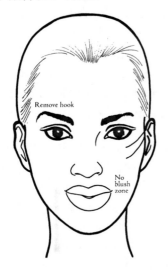

Remove hook

No
blush
zone

You have a slim, delicate structure. Start your blusher placement at the outer edge of the apple. Keep color on the cheekbone toward the top. Make wide sweeps toward the upper part of ear and hairline.

You want to create optical and aesthetic horizontal lines of color to suggest width. Don't shade or contour the temples, jaw-line, or chin. Color in the center zone of the face is important. Eyebrows should be on a horizontal plane, with a high center arch. Eye shadow is earthy, gold, topaz, peachy-red, soft berry; no brown-black or black outer corner shading. Lip pencil liner emphasizes, broadens, and plays up full lips. Apply color to the very edge.

Special Blusher Tips

For the ultimate, long-lasting glow, apply a cream blusher over your foundation and set it with translucent powder. Then apply a complementary powder blusher over the translucent face powder and blend. You will have a day-long natural glow.

With or without make-up, daily skin care is a must. Here, these lovely ladies have enhanced their natural beauty with the appropriate base and colors that contour.

Your Fabulous Lips

The most attractive part of an African-American women's face is her lips. No one smiles with such full lips and with such beautiful white teeth. The secure black woman who really believes that black is beautiful has no problem accepting God's gift. She flaunts her full lips when talking with a friend, communicating at work, attending religious affairs, flirting, or just being sensual.

A black woman has a natural, firm, raised lip line. The natural pout in the center and her thick upper and lower lips are attractive. Learn how to express your lovely features by practicing before a mirror. Maximize the value and beauty of your lips. But be honest with yourself, too. If your lips have droopy, turned-down corners, teach yourself to hold the corners up. Smile more and practice looking pleasant.

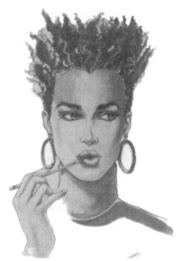

Besides how you hold your lips, your mouth may have other "spoilers" needing attention—for example, missing teeth, gold teeth, yellow teeth, or poorly manufactured partial dentures. Your lips dramatically outline your mouth, therefore your teeth must not be a major negative to an otherwise beautiful face. When you have moist, dewy, luscious lips, your teeth in their whiteness and evenness only make you more inviting. Your lips, teeth, and smile make your face radiate, bringing joy to all who see you.

Lip Color Options

If you are a woman who prefers just a hint of natural color (earth tones to soft beige, or pink tones), I have a suggestion: even out discolorations with concealer or your foundation base and set with powder. If your upper and lower lips are dark and even, for best results select a lip shade lighter than your lips.

You might wish to apply a lipstick product from a tube, wand, pan, or pot. There are lip glosses designed for women of color—deeply pigmented shades that can be worn alone; they impart a moist, sheer sheen to your lips. Or you might wish to wear a clear lip gloss or lip moisturizer. This, too, would be appropriate. Don't use greasy, nonpenetrating petroleum jelly, however. It looks and feels tacky on your lips. You might want to take the time to use a lip pencil, for it is excellent in achieving a natural look. If you use a lip pencil, lightly line the lip and fill in with the pencil, covering any uneven tones, then apply a clear red, a brown lip shade, or clear tint gloss.

If you are conservative but want a pulled-together look, I suggest the medium-tone creams (clear red, russet-red, radiant red, cocoa-copper, cinnamon, café, brandied coral, raspberry, spice sienna, and so on).

Dark skin usually looks best in shades of beige, yellow, yellow-brown, and blue. For example, if you are of medium tone with yellow-brown skin and a sallow aura, lipsticks with a beige or deep yellow base will drain color from your skin. On the other hand, you can wear deep orange shades such as cinnamon-orange, burnt orange, radiant red, bronze-coral) and claret.

Lipstick Tools

Now let's consider the lipstick tools and materials: lip liner pencil, lip brush, lip light, lip toner or foundation, and lip balancer.

1. **Lip Liner Pencil**. Liner pencils define the line of the lips and should be chosen with your skin tone in mind. For example, if you have fair to light skin) your liner should be rose-pink, light red, light plum, or light brown. Women with medium skin tones are best using liner pencils in shades of red, light brown, brown, and plum. Those with dark skin tones look best using red, deep brown, raspberry, plum, or brown-black liners. **Never** use a black pencil to line your lips. It's unattractive and appears harsh.

   When you want a new look for your lips, use a lip pencil. Lightly outline the lips and fill in the corners if your lips are full, and then edge in your selected color. The pencil should match as closely as possible to the desired lip color.

Some women have deep folds in their lips that extend to the outer edges. Lip color frequently cakes and peels to these edges, giving the appearance of bleeding color. The lip liner pencil keeps lip color from bleeding and gives a more precise lip line. When matte, oil-free pencils are used as a base for cream or frosted lipsticks, the color stays put and wears much longer.

2. **Lip Brush**. The purpose of a lipstick brush is to transfer lipstick from the tube to the surface of the lips in a smooth application. The brush gets color into the crevices as well, giving a smooth, full-color application. The lipstick brush also gives you the option of lining your lips (see previous item), reducing the possibility of your lipstick bleeding once the large area is colored.

   A lipstick brush may be either man-made, of natural fibers, or a combination of both. I recommend a blend of natural and man-made fibers.

3. **Lip Light**. Lip light is a lip color adjuster, which reflects light colors away from ruddy, bluish, or very dark lips; it is worn under the lipstick.

4. **Lip Toner**. A lip toner, or foundation, is a lip adjuster that corrects slightly discolored lips, evens out lip tones, and keeps color true. Toners come in fair-to-medium and medium-to-dark shades.

5. **Lip Balancer**. A lip balancer is a deep, waxy, purplish teak natural pigment, designed to camouflage the resistant light pink discoloration often found on medium and dark lips. A lip balancer also neutralizes the acidity that causes discoloration in the center of the bottom lip, an area which is more often affected than the upper. In the process, it prevents the lipstick from changing color when placed on this area. A lip balancer is worn under the lipstick. It is excellent for subtle, medium, and deep shades of lipstick; however, the bright reds, orange-browns, and light berry shades are affected by a lip balancer.

Types of Lipstick

Lipstick types are very personal preferences, and it is up to you which you select. Lipsticks with specially formulated conditioners, moisturizers, waxes, and light mineral oil are superior to those without them, since these ingredients smooth the lips, help retain moisture, help prevent infection, and often protect sensitive skin.

Here's a special beauty note: most lipstick formulas include conditioners and emollients. For example, lip moisturizers often contain PABA (a sunscreen) along with vitamins A and E. So there are advantages over and above beauty for using a lipstick.

Now, let's review some of the major types of lipstick available today:

1. **Cream Lipsticks**. Standard cream lipsticks are deep pigment colors without shine. They wear longer and impart more coverage than the noncream sticks owing to their heavy wax base. A second cream formula is more lightweight in texture and does not feel as heavy on the lips, but it also does not wear as long because it usually has a mineral oil base.

2. **Frosted Lipsticks**. Frosted lipsticks are usually heavy pigment colors with an iridescent, pearlized, or opaque gold coverage. Women of color look best in iridescent gold eye shadow, highlights, blusher highlights in gold, and most certainly lipsticks with a gold or yellow base.

3. **Silver Sparkling Frost**. Silver sparkling frost usually looks ridiculous if applied to dark or very dark skin. This is because it imparts an ashy gray look to red-brown or bluish brown skin undertones.

4. **Long-lasting Lipsticks**. There are lipsticks formulated to last far longer than regular lipsticks. New research and development has produced long-wearing, non-smear lipstick formulas approved for women of color.

5. **Matte Lipsticks**. No-shine lipstick formulas have conditioners for a non-dry look and feel.

6. **Translucent Lipsticks.** Translucent lipsticks in tubes or wands impart just a hint of color, with sheer coverage.

7. **Lip Glosses.** Glosses have a clear, shiny, transparent base. They come in pans, pots, wands, and tubes. Some have conditioners and moisturizers, and claim healing properties. They are usually worn over lipstick to impart a sheer gloss. Lip glosses can be worn alone, as well.

8. **Nonfragrance Lipsticks.** Fragrance-free lipsticks are for sensitive and acne skin. When some women have an allergic swelling, or experience an itchy, burning sensation on their lips, this may be a reaction to their lipstick. Most women sensitive to lipstick are reacting to the lanolin, fragrance, dyes, or preservatives in the formula. If this is a problem for you, buy fragrance-free, dermatologically tested, hypoallergenic lipstick.

Applying Lip Color

The lip brush is used to pick up a small amount of lip color, and then to outline the lips, filling in from the center of the mouth to the outer edges. The following is the procedure I suggest for having beautifully colored lips:

1. Apply a lip color adjuster, such as lip light.

2. Outline your lips with a sharp lip liner pencil.

3. Edge in the lipstick color along the pencil outline and coat the lips, starting with the bottom and moving to the upper lip. Apply more color in the center, moving outward to the edges. If your lips are smooth, apply color directly from the tube.

4. Add lip gloss for a moist effect or gleam.

See the illustrations that follow for specific techniques.

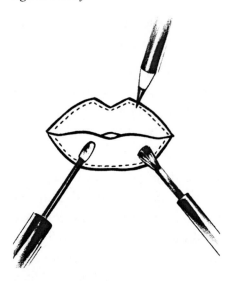

Full, puckered lips with lines. Your full lips usually have an attractive ridge that gives them a definite lip line. Cover your lips with foundation, preferably an oil-free formula. Blot with oil-free setting powder.

Most of us have lined, curved, crinkly lips. For best results, edge in a faint lip line with a lip brush or a lip pencil hay a shade darker (light and medium brown, red, and berry hues) for aesthetic illusions. Follow with a lip brush to produce a smooth appearance; gently stretch your lips with your index finger and draw in a smooth line. Top lip brush with gloss.

Thin lips. Cover the lips and edges with foundation. Set with oil-free powder. Redefine the lip shape you want with a lip liner pencil in a shade darker than your selected lipstick color. Fill in with lipstick and add a touch of gloss to give a moist, dewy appearance.

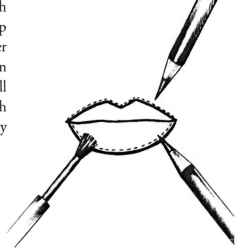

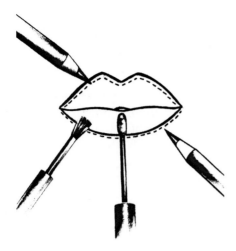

When one lip is larger than the other, apply foundation over the larger lip, set with oil-free powder, then edge in a line inside your natural lip line with a pencil or brush. Fill in with lipstick. Now follow the natural lip line of the smaller lip with a pencil or brush, and fill in with lipstick.

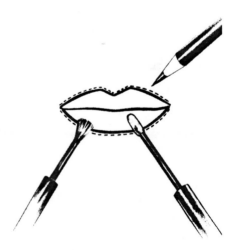

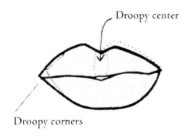

Droopy center

Droopy corners

Unbalanced and droopy lips. Cover the lips with foundation, and set with oil-free powder. Balance the uneven lip portion by straightening the lip line with a pencil, using a shade darker than your selected lipstick color. Blot with powder. Fill in with lipstick color.

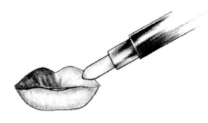

To balance a droopy center, apply medium shade of oil-free concealer vertically through the center of the droop. Outline with pencil and lip brush, and fill in with lipstick. To cover the natural lip line at the corner, edge in with a medium dark oil-free cover stick. Blot with powder.

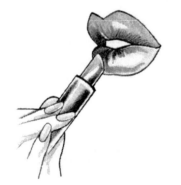

To lift a corner to create an optical illusion, use a lip pencil to extend the lower lip, taking the line upward. Continue the line just a bit above the upper lip corner. Now, extend the upper lip line to meet it. Blot with powder and fill in with lipstick color. Use a pencil, impossible.

Discolored lips. You have four options:

1. Use lip light to reflect light evenly away from uneven dark lips.

2. Use oil-free lip toner or foundation to even out lip color.

3. Use lip balancer as a natural stain to even out acid buildup on the pink discoloration. Lip balancer will interfere with light lipstick shade,.

4. Use a medium to dark oil-free cover stick to help even out discolored lips.

Dry, crinkly, lined lips. Condition lips with gloss or lip moisturizer which contains mineral oil, cocoa butter, phenol, alum, camphor, and beeswax.

Five-Minute Face
The following order of make-up application should be followed:

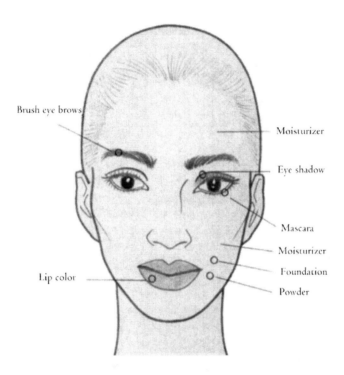

1. Moisturize
2. Add foundation
3. Set foundation with powder
4. Do eyes: one color eyelid and eye color application
5. Apply mascara
6. Brush eyebrows
7. Add lipstick color

Ten-Minute Face

Use the following order to apply make-up:

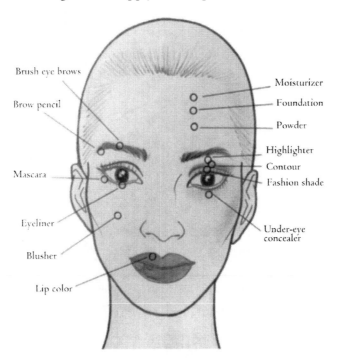

1. Moisturize
2. Add foundation
3. Apply powder to set foundation
4. Do eyes: apply eye concealer, highlight brow bone with color, contour center of eyelid with color; apply fashion eye color to area closest to eyelash; apply eye liner, mascara; brush eyebrow and apply brow pencil
5. Apply blusher
6. Apply lip color

Fifteen-Minute Face
Use the following order to apply make-up:

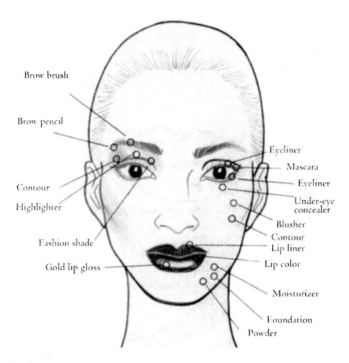

Brow brush

Brow pencil

Contour

Highlighter

Fashion shade

Gold lip gloss

Eyeliner

Mascara

Eyeliner

Under-eye concealer

Blusher

Contour

Lip liner

Lip color

Moisturizer

Foundation

Powder

1. Moisturize

2. Apply under-eye concealer

3. Apply foundation

4. Apply powder to set foundation

5. Do eyes: for rainbow eyes, apply fashion shade to under corner of eye, highlight the center point of eyelid, contour the outer corner of eyelid; apply eyeliner to top and bottom lid; use brow brush, brow pencil, mascara

6. Do cheeks: contour the cheek area underneath the cheekbone and then apply blusher on top of cheekbone, blending down to contour

7. Do lips: use lip pencil to line lips, add lip color with lip brush, and add a touch of lip gloss

Viva la difference—before and after!

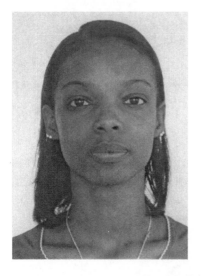 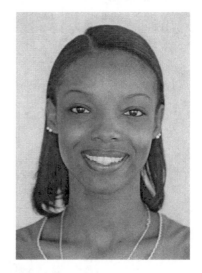

Karima Henderson, Career Girl

Color Plan: Rich Copper foundation with a deep shade of pressed powder, Earth-tone eye shadows in red-brown and salmon, with black eyeliner pencil and soft black mascara, Rose blusher, and red lipstick.

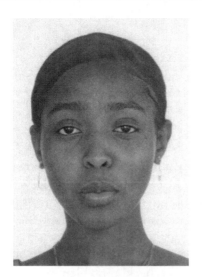 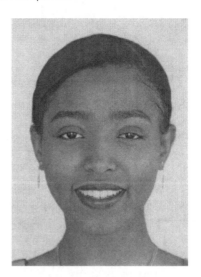

Rabiya Dumas, College Student

Color Plan: Deep Bronze foundation with powder, Smoky Bronze and Medium Tan eyeshadow, with black eyeliner and mascara, Rustique blusher, and Russet Red lipstick.

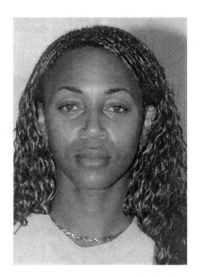 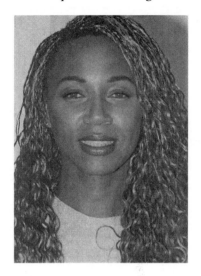

Lena Nicholson, Flight Attendant

Color Plan: Mocha-brown foundation with powder, Bold Brown and Smoky Grey eyeshadow with blue-black liner and mascara, Deep Red blusher, and Royal Red lipstick.

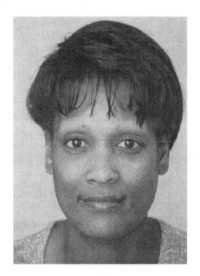 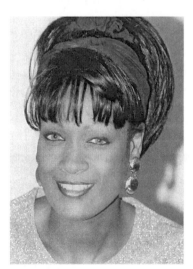

Cindy Gabbidon, Model

Color Plan: Amber foundation with powder, Soft Rose and Smoky Brown eyeshadow, with brown-black eyeliner and soft black mascara, Hot Pink blusher, and Fuchsia lipstick.

Teen Talk...Special Things To Remember

The Flair for Color

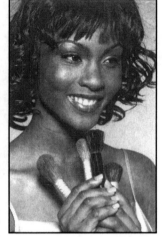

Teenagers of color are born to wear unusual colors in every hue: Royal Purple, Mysterious Black, Exciting Red, Romantic Pink, Peach and Lavender and Earthy Coppers, Red-Orange, Terra-Cotta, Orange, Tan, Brown, and Gold.

Now let's learn how to combine colors and select shades that will make the most of your facial beauty – your eyes, skin and hair. No need to take out a loan from your parents and spend all of your disposable money on makeup and hair. Color is what's happening.

Teenagers of color are on the move. Your presence and your beauty have left a mark in women's sports, music, dance, religion, acting, fashion and education, and will continue to do so as you continue to daringly break the color rules. So keep up the good work!

Special Stuff

Eye shadow comes in dozens of colors, including pearlescent, matte, crème and satin textures. For a special night out, touch a little to your cheeks to create face-flattering accents or try a little pearlescent eye shadow on the tips of your lashes for a fabulous flutter.

Teen Tips:

Smart and Sensible Suggestions

o   The best suggestion for a teenage girl regarding your personal beauty regimen is: wear makeup that looks natural and that is age appropriate for your group.

o   It is most unattractive when a teen shaves off her eyebrows and then uses eyebrow pencil to draw in a line. This gives your face a severe look. So, don't shave the eyebrow off and then put a new one on. Instead, shape or fill in your existing eyebrow.

Mascara:

Your curly lashes look thick and luxurious. If you don't have enough curl, here's how you get it. Look directly into a mirror. Take a lash curler, open it, and bring it right up toward your eye. Secure your lashes between the rubber grips and squeeze for about fifteen seconds. *Voila!* Curly lashes, ready to coat with your favorite color mascara!

Use Blushers with Moderation

The ideal application should create only a suggestion, or hint of color. Select rich, pure colors, such as copper-bronze with its deep gold base, or a soft plum, light wine-burgundy, or a deeply pigmented almond-orange shade. When you apply powder blusher, always dip the brush quickly and flick or twist your wrist to stroke the cheek lightly. Remember: it is better to apply just a little blusher and then go back and apply more if you need it, than to apply too much and have to disturb the foundation to remove the excess. Matte colors (no shine) are best for day-time on all skin types.

Blushers can do more to add warmth and radiance than any other cosmetics We feature the following four basic face shapes; however, different faces require different techniques. If your face shape is not here, combine the features from others to obtain the right techniques.

To find your face shape, tie your hair up and away from your face and look into the mirror. If you still can't tell, get a ruler and measure your forehead from temple to temple, cheekbone to cheekbone and jawline to jawline. Place measurements on paper and connect with rounded lines.

Annoying Allergies

There are a host of various cosmetics with different ingredients. If a teen experiences itching or redness, or bumps from her makeup, then use of that makeup should be discontinued immediately. You should not try another makeup until the rash symptoms resolve completely. Then you can read the list of ingredients and find a different makeup type that does not have that ingredient in it.

An allergy is a reaction of the body to a foreign material that it tries to reject or forms a reaction to it. Allergies can come from various foods, particularly shellfish and nuts. In terms of cosmetics, allergies can come from hair dyes, particularly black hair dyes that contain a chemical phenylenediamine, which commonly causes allergies. Nail polishes and lacquers contain formaldehydes that can cause allergic reactions not only on the hands, but particularly around the eyes. Eyeliner, mascara and contact lens solution can all cause allergies on the skin.

Beauty Note—Love Your Lips

The dark upper lip is a beautiful contrast to the healthy pink bottom lip, or vice versa. Do what actresses and supermodels of color do: treat your lips as a beauty asset. Flaunt those full lips with plum, brown, mocha, cinnamon, or red lip liner pencil. Then apply clear or colored lip gloss, starting from the corners in toward the center of your lips.

Let's Review!! The Ultra-Grand Makeup Application

Here we suggest the appropriate makeup steps to maintain your warm, healthy youthful appeal:

Start with a clean, fresh face.

Step One - Foundation
Tool - Makeup Sponge

Concealer is applied to the entire eyelid to serve as a foundation for eye shadow (shadow stays in place longer and appears to be smoother) and under-eye area to give a smoother effect and conceal uneven, blotchy skin tones. A damp sponge is preferred (a dry sponge lifts too much foundation). Place foundation on uneven parts of the face and fill in. Blend and then observe. If necessary, cover the entire face. Final movement should be light, downward strokes. (Set your foundation with translucent powder. If your skin is very dry to extremely dry, powder is optional).

Step Two - Eye Shadow
Tool - Eye makeup applicator

Movements – highlight brow bone. Contour center of eye to give the concave effect and finally apply the fashion color closest to the eyelash area. Blend and set with powder.

Step Three - Eyeliner
Tool - Eyeliner Pencil, liquid or cake powder liner

Should be applied close to the lashes, drawing line from inner to outer corners.

Step Four - Brows
Tool - Brow comb and brush, brow gel, cake powder brush-on-brow, and pencil.

Fill in brow pencil or cake powder and comb or brush back into shape. If hairs are unruly, apply brow gel. If gel is tinted, apply and brush.

Step Five - Eyelashes
Tool - Eyelash wand

Apply lash-building, waterproof, or sensitive formula mascara. Stroke up and out. If lashes are extremely curly, hold wand vertically, as demonstrated, and swing left to right, hitting the tips of the lashes.

Step Six - Blush
Tool - Blush brush

Apply blush to cheek bone area. Move along cheek area outward to the hairline.

Step Seven - Lips
Tool - Lip brush, lip pencil, lip liner

Apply lipstick with a brush to fill in the grooves or lines on lips or lip lines with lip liner for shaping, add color to discolored lip with pencil, and fill in with lip color and gloss.

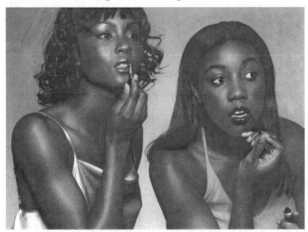

Quiz: Adding Color to Your Face

Q. Where do you start adding blusher?
A. Use the outer corner of your eye as a guide to start adding blusher

Q. What skin type should use powder eye shadow?
A. Powder eye shadow is good for all skin types

Q. What zone do you avoid when applying blusher?
A. Never apply blusher to the "no blush zone" between the apple of your cheekbone and the bloom of your nose.

Q. What should you do when you want to test mascara in the store?
A. Always ask the makeup artist for a clean wand to prevent the spread of bacteria.

Q. In which direction should you apply blusher/
A. Always move across, upward and out toward the hairline.

Q. What lipstick shades would you wear to get a hint of natural color?
A. Try lipsticks in earth tones to soft beige or pink tones.

Q. Should you add blusher underneath your eyes?
A. No, do not add blusher underneath eyes near the lower rim.

Q. What is a matte color?
A. A color with no shine.

Beauty Note

Your lips suffer in the winter. Use a mineral oil lip preparation to trap and seal moisture on your lips. Medicated formulas relieve cracking, peeling, bleeding and splitting.

Ask Mercedes Fleetwood

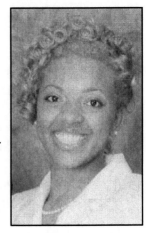

When choosing makeup colors, do I choose colors that compliment my complexion or my outfit?

Actually, you should try to do both – your complexion should dictate the depth of the color you use and your outfit should dictate the tone. Earthtones are usually safest and there are many shades of brown that you can choose for starters. Save the rainbow colors for those glamorous outfits in shades of purple, blue and green – but take care not to wear light colors that may look too ashy on your skin or bright colors that may look overstated or sleazy. When you are not sure, the rule of thumb is 'less is best'.

Chapter 7

Your Hair, Hands, and Nails

The Right Hairstyle

Today's salon hairstylists are a refreshing new breed of creative, skill-ful, talented people who can make appropriate suggestions concerning your hair care, as well as cut, curl, and style your hair—all based on your facial shape.

If you consider working with your hair, keep your face in mind. Too much hair moving forward toward the center of your head, with bangs falling into your eyes will show age on your face more than any other hairstyle; hair moving away from the center of your forehead takes years off your face.

If you have a low forehead and a short neck, you can give the illusion of adding more height by styling your hair high, with medium curls on your head, and by keeping your hair away from your neck, styling it close to the sides of your head. On the other hand, when a woman's hair is long, all anyone sees is her head and shoulders; they don't see her neck. If your neck is long and you have a high forehead, style your hair to fall into soft curls, some to the side and some across the forehead in a sculptured fashion.

To give you some styling ideas, I have put together a collection of hairstyles that address problems with the neck, forehead, nose, jaw, and chin. These styles vary from straight or curly cuts to corn rows. They are to excite your imagination while providing the necessary clues you can employ to camouflage a problem.

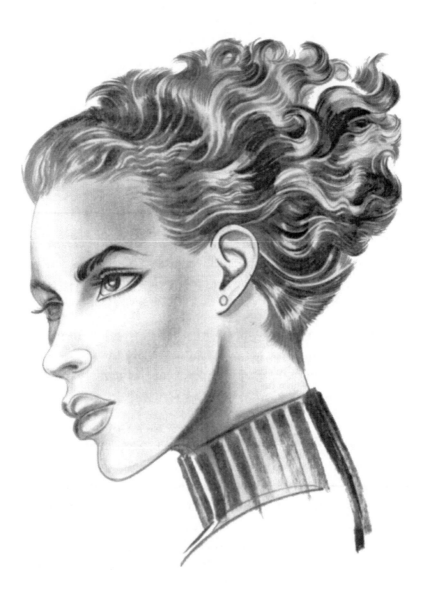

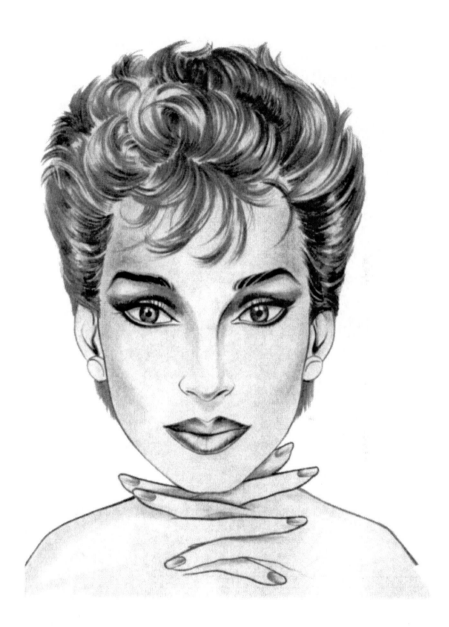

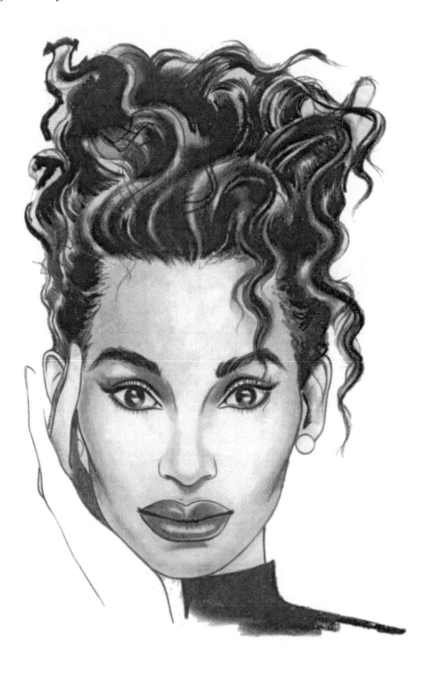

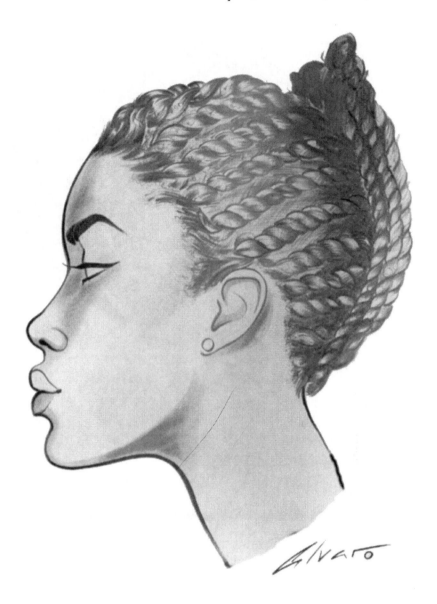

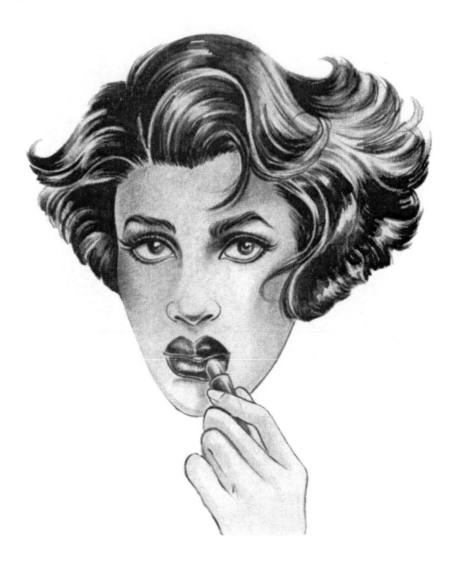

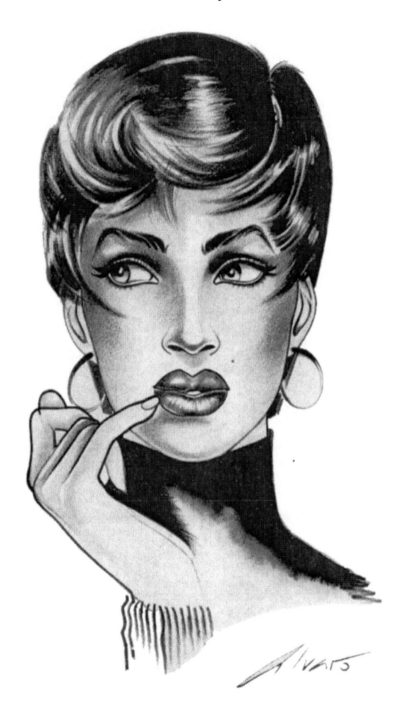

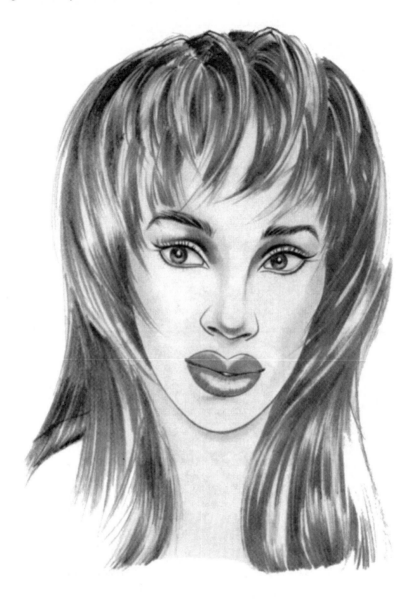

Hair Shaping

The right haircut and shape is the key to an ideal hairstyle. Women must go regularly to a professional beauty salon for shaping and cutting. Some women prefer a barber shop, but I recommend a women's salon. The lines and symmetry for women's hairstyles are entirely different from men's.

In cutting and shaping your hair, a professional should take your features and facial shape into consideration. Extreme hairstyles are not for you.

Hair Color

When I was beauty editor at *Ebony* magazine, the editors of *Chain and Drug Store* magazine, a trade publication, asked me, "What were the newest trends in hair grooming products for the black woman of the '90s?" The answer was obvious: the African-American woman wanted more color in her life. Black women wanted to enhance and highlight their otherwise very dark hair. Well, what was perceived as a trend then is now an avalanche. I could not be happier. Today's black woman of the millennium is throwing off the shackles of dowdy conservatism and using color.

No longer is it just black companies that are preparing hair products for blacks. Clairol's innovative Instant Water conditioning beauty shampoo-in formula and Dark and Lovely's conditioning formulas, and Revlon's Color Style Tints are excellent examples of what is happening in the retail market. My favorite new hair colorings are the fabulous berry shades that range from strawberry to plum. And the rich bronzes and browns with apricot-cinnamon and chestnut highlights are fabulous, and some blondes do have more fun, too. Variety is definitely here!

Like your skin undertone, your hair has a tone that ranges from yellow-gold or yellow-red to red, dark red, or red-brown, and to brown-black. Your skin tone, eye color, and natural hair color are great guides in choosing a correct hair color. Remember: you have my color chart in the photo insert to help you. You also have help available from your beauty-salon hair colorist and the manufacturer's information in the insert and on the back of the hair coloring package.

The best guide to choosing a hair color, however, is a hair strand test, which you can do yourself. Test a strand or section of hair to see how the new color will relate to your eyes and skin. Also determine how the change makes you feel—before going all the way. Take a strand from underneath your outer layer of hair so it won't show if you decide not to proceed. The strand test can be done under the supervision of your hair colorist or at home with an over-the-counter product.

Whichever coloring process you choose—home or salon—there are three basic types of hair color:

Temporary color

These are shampoo-in formulas that are nonalkaline and work gently with the natural chemistry of your hair. Temporary colors are noncoating and will not penetrate the hair shaft. Temporary colors wash out, and usually do not contain ammonia, peroxide, or other harmful ingredients.

Semipermanent color

These are designed to harden and coat the outer cuticle shaft of the hair. Semipermanent colors start to rinse off after four or six washings. Some semipermanent color products contain peroxide.

Permanent color

These change the character pigment balance and natural hair color. Permanent hair coloring is best applied in a salon by a professional hair colorist, particularly if you are insecure about your first color change. Permanent hair color products last longer than any other hair change process. Special care for treated or relaxed hair is advised.

Color crayons

"Tween-Time Hair" and "Cover Gray" are excellent touch-up tools, made of tea, stearate, paraffin, and beeswax. Hair coloring crayons are designed to conceal the roots of your natural hair growth between temporary, semipermanent, and permanent hair colorings. You moisten the crayon and apply it to the hair shaft.

There are other natural and synthetic ways to change your hair color, including special formulas to cover gray hair, color tints, color sprays, mousses, natural henna, and comb-in hair coloring.

Your Hands Are Lovely

Lovely hands can be the ultimate statement in your total grooming regimen. But making that statement requires proper care.

Your hands are constantly exposed to stresses: weather, pollutants, detergents and other irritating chemicals, and dirt. They get cut, bruised and scraped. When you clean your hands, you usually wash them in soap and water, removing the limited moisture and oils the body has provided to protect them. Your hands do not have as many oil producing glands or as much fatty tissue per square inch as does your face. There are no oil glands on the palms of your hands (sweat glands, yes). Thus, washing with drying soaps is more stressful for your hands than you probably realize.

Often, the results of poor hand care can be seen in the ashen-colored skin between the thumb and index finger, and on the knuckles and cuticles of many women. Regardless of your skin tone, dry-looking skin is unattractive. It shows up more on dark skin, and therefore requires a more intensive hand-care regimen. As you would suppose, the seasons of the year affect your hands differently, and the worst season is winter.

Winter hand care usually means applying an extra-dry hand-cream formula. I do not recommend petroleum jelly, since it gives the hands a greasy, tacky look and feel. It also attracts dirt, particles to the hands and under the nails. There are excellent over-the-counter hand-care products to use, but you must use them faithfully.

Proper care of the hands also requires periodic, regular pampering, which includes a regular manicure. Learn from your manicurist and care for your hands personally between visits.

Your Nails and Their Care

Let's look at some important terms before discussing nail health and care. The nail mantle is a protective plate located at the end of the finger. It is made up of the following:

1. The nail bed upon which the nail surface rests.

2. The cuticle, a thin outer layer of the nail skin epidermis.

3. The matrix, or formative intercellular tissue of the nail; blood cells nourish the matrix.

4. The lunula, or whitish half-moon shape at the base of the fingernail. The important, often-abused cuticles serve to protect the nail and keep environmental impurities and germs away from the healthy growing nail.

Nail-Care Products and Processes

There are several terms that a manicurist uses in caring for your nails.

o **Nail bleach**—a salon manicuring cosmetic used to remove stains from under the edges of the fingernail tips.

o **Nail white**—a nail cosmetic used to whiten the free edge of the nail.

o **Nail white pencil**—a pencil containing a hard white chalk, used to whiten the free edge underneath the fingernail tips.

o **Nail enamel or polish**—a fingernail polish in the form of a liquid, which forms a colored or transparent coating on glued-on fingernails.

o **Nail lacquer**—a thick liquid that forms a high glossy film on your nails.

o **Nail transplants**—process by which a manicurist cements a broken fingernail to a natural nail.

o **Nail extensions**—process by which a manicurist applies a pre-mixed material at the juncture of the natural fingernail tip and the silver-foil nail form, forming and sculpturing an artificially extended nail.

o   **Nail wrappings**—process by which the manicurist covers the nail's outer tissue, sealing it with a protective nail enamel or glaze, for a smoother, harder, and more durable nail prepared to receive enamel.

Artificial Nails

Any health care provider experienced with hand and nail care will agree that artificial nails cause all kinds of problems for nails. Fungus infections and bacterial growth is a major concern.

Nail Health

A healthy nail grows 1/32 of an inch each week. Nails grow rapidly until you are 30, and then as you mature their growth rate decreases to one half the youthful rate. Of course, a good diet, regular exercise, and adequate water consumption will enhance the health of your nails.

Slower than normal nail growth can result in excessive thickening of the nails. Breaking, splitting, and peeling can be hereditary or can result from a dietary deficiency or nutritional imbalance. If any of these conditions worsen, consult your physician or dermatologist before your next manicure.

Also, if at any time you notice that your hands show a reddish-yellowing, with a reddish purple aura against a white background, immediately consult your doctor.

Likewise, if you have infected, sensitive crusty dark cuticles, swollen and sensitive skin at the sides of the nails and fingertips, skin discolorations, or rashes and fine bumps, you should be concerned and seek medical advice.

Home Care of Your Nails

The use of chemicals, internal and topical medications, drastic diet changes, and nail color, polish removers, artificial nails, and nail base coats can often cause nail discoloration, nail breakage, dryness, and general poor nail health. If possible, wear gloves when working in the garden, washing dishes, and so on. Buff your nails on occasion, giving them a relief from the nail base and polish. Be careful with your eating habits and don't go on crash diets. Watch your medication; don't be pill happy, as so many of us are. Good nutrition and proper vitamin supplements will help keep your nails healthy while doing wonders for your entire system.

Regularly consult a professional manicurist. Ask your manicurist to teach you how to care for your hands and nails in between visits.

Teen Talk...Special Things To Remember

Make Your Hairstyle Unique

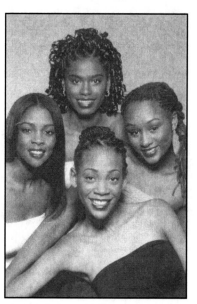

There's so much to know about your hair. During your lifetime, you will probably wear a number of different styles and lengths, and perhaps even a number of different colors.

In people of color, there have been eighteen different hair follicle types noted, which come in coarse, medium and fine textures. For a great look, the challenge is to find your own best style. Look for a style that complements your face shape. Look in a mirror, pull your hair back and check it out:

- o **Oblong.** Your chin is long and your forehead is high. Choose soft, rounded styles, which do not lengthen your face. One such method is to have a feathery bang. Hair looks best at jaw length, full and off the face. If you decide to wear your hair long, avoid a straight look.

- o **Oval.** This face is balanced, with chin and forehead about the same size. Lucky you! Oval is considered to be the perfect model shape. Just about any hairstyle will fit the oval face's features. Choose a style that best suits your hair texture and type. Your choices can include bobs, braids, weaves, curls, waves, or straight looks.

- o **Round.** This face shape is rather full, especially at the cheeks. You should build as much height as possible with your hair – this will give you the look of length to your face. Avoid framing your face with too much hair, particularly with thickness at ear length. Clean, straight lines will contour and slenderize your face. An excellent choice for a round face is a bob cut.

o **Square**. Your forehead and jawline are both broad and almost the same width. If you have a square face, you should soften the lines, both on your forehead and chin, by having your hair fall gently to those areas. Asymmetrical styles, layered cuts, or soft waves work well to flatter the squareness of your face.

o **Heart**. Your forehead and cheeks will be the widest parts of the face, which gets narrowed at the chin. For a heart-shaped face, you may opt to wear a flip with a soft cropped bang. This will give an illusion of fullness in your cheek area.

o **Pear**. Your jawline and cheeks are fuller than your forehead. To add balance to a pear-shaped face, wear your hair short and full. Keep it cropped at ear length for best results.

Special Stuff

There might be some beauty schools in your area where young fashion-forward stylists, working to complete their class credits, need to work on models. This could be a great way to get your new look, without paying an arm and a leg for it.

The 411 About Hairstyles You May be Considering

Hair Weaves, Braids and Extensions

These alternatives include getting a full weave, braids or just a few tracks to add fullness and length to your own hair. For those of you who have not tried either technique, here are a few details:

Full Weaves

A full weave is done on your entire head in either of two methods. This is the most popular. All your natural hair can be cornrowed in a flat braid around your entire head. Wefts of hair are then sewn onto the tracks in the best direction to fall into the shape that you desire. (You can choose any texture, quality, color or length of hair – preferably human hair). Once all of the hair is sewn on, it will be cut and styled as you wish.

Interlocking

This is a form of braiding, but it resembles a weave. Your natural hair is braided individually, with hair extensions mixed in, then locked or knitted close to the scalp. This looks very natural – the hair remains loose or full, creating a weave look. (Always use human hair for this technique).

Braids

There are so many styles to choose from. Have fun with this in a style that's long or short – braids that are thick or thin, loose and long, or cornrowed and contoured. Synthetic hair is best for braided styles – again choose your favorite color.

Natural Styles

If your hair is naturally curly, why straighten it with chemicals? Wear it with pride. And those short Afros are quite chic too; but the loc is growing in trendiness. Locs are a fashion statement unto themselves.

Whether it's for spiritual reasons, as an affirmation of power, or just plain fashion sense, if you opt for locs you're a brave little sister. The process of loc'ing the hair takes about three to six months. During this time, your hair will go through several stages, some very difficult to manage. For best results, you should get it started professionally by a loctician. Every few months thereafter, treat yourself to a professional grooming to make sure that your hair is cleaned thoroughly and properly conditioned. Between appointments, however, be sure to clean and moisturize your hair and scalp regularly.

Straightened Hair

By taking the curl or kink out of your hair, it will become straightened, which will greatly expand your styling choices. Before chemical relaxers were developed, everyone straightened (pressed) their hair with a pressing comb and then curled it with a curling iron or set it on rollers. But, of course, this had to be done every time your hair was shampooed. I do believe that before chemical relaxers were developed, hair was much healthier and maintained its thickness much longer. Today, chemical straightening is quicker and lasts much longer, but your poor hair suffers. Overprocessing and underconditioning are the two biggest culprits.

Chemical relaxers are the most popular method of hair straightening and the most important step toward getting the style of your choice, but you are cautioned to use care. Know your stylist, or if you do it yourself, read and follow the directions completely. Once you have relaxed your hair, you can usually get the cut or shape that you want. Enjoy!

Hair's the Facts
- Your hair grows about half an inch a month.
- Don't worry if you see a little shedding when you comb. Hair sheds too, just like skin does when you bathe.
- Regular trims are okay and they keep the splits away.

Best Tools for Styling Your Hair

o   Natural boar bristle brushes are good if you wear your hair natural or if it has been chemically treated. They won't snag and break your hair like brushes with nylon or synthetic bristles.

o   Rubber bristle brushes with large round tips are good if your hair is weaved.

o   Combs are for detangling or smoothing your hair. Wide-tooth rubber combs are unquestionable the preferred tool for you. They also work well for combing conditioner through your hair while you are in the shower.

o   Picks are good for natural hair. If you are wearing an Afro, or if your hair is very curly, a pick is a must-have.

Those Little Extras

o Barrettes	o Coated Rubber Hair Bands
o Bobby Pins	o Hair Clips
o Hair Pins	o Clip on Hairpieces
o Headbands	o Sparkles

Blow Dryers

Whatever type of blow dryer fits your hands best can work. Be sure that you don't have the heat too high if your hair is chemically processed.

Curlers and Straightening Combs

o If you want to change your straight hairstyle pronto, curl the ends with an electric curling iron. Watch that heat, though.

o Rollers that use steam are great for keeping the moisture in your hair, if you've got the time to sit for a while.

o Plastic or metal rollers work well for a wet set, but always use end papers first, to keep ends from catching or breaking.

o Straightening combs are available in electric or stove-top styles. In both cases, watch the temperature – these will burn your hair if they get too hot.

Hair Care Supplies

o Shampoo (alternate between those with and without built-in conditioners).

o Instant conditioners for regular weekly or biweekly shampoos.

o Deep-penetrating conditioners with protein or other natural ingredients for one or two treatments per month.

o Hair moisturizer or oil for daily scalp treatment and hair grooming.

o Hair gel for quick slick looks.

o Hair mousse for fun full styles.

o Hair spray to keep it all together.

Your Glorious Nails – They Can Be Even More Beautiful!

Lovely hands can be the ultimate statement in your total grooming regimen. But making that statement requires proper care.

Hand Exam: Can You Positively Answer Yes to These Questions?

1. Are your nails uniformly shaped and in proportionate lengths?

2. Are your nails healthy – minus splits and breaks?

3. Are your nails neatly manicured?

4. Are your knuckles soft and smooth?

5. Are your hands soft and supple on both the outer side and the palms?

Smart and Sensible Suggestions for You

o When you go to a manicurist, take your own tools with you, such as: *manicure orangewood sticks, nail clipper, cuticle shaper, cuticle trimmer, scissors, buffer. You may even prefer to use your own, base coat polish and top coat.* Buy everything and keep it in a little pouch. Then take it with you. This will help decrease the spread of infection.

o Artificial nails are fine for special occasions, you just don't want to wear them for long periods of time. If you're addicted to them, you need to take them off at least every three months or so to give your nails a rest. Prolonged use can lead to thinning of the nails and fungus and you can never regain your former strong nails.

o When choosing nail polish colors, remember that clear or neutral shades don't show up chips as much as brighter or darker colors. Shimmery, sparkly nail polish is great but all your nail flaws will show. Also, the lighter your polish, the longer your nails look.

Planning to do your own manicures at home? To help you care for your nails, here's a basic at home program. You will need a bowl of warm sudsy water, a bowl of clear water and towels….. Also, assemble the following:

1. **Polish remover** – a fragrance-free, oil-based formula without acetone.

2. **Nail file** – wood or metal for shaping and cleaning.

3. **Cream or liquid cuticle remover** – aids in the removal of dead skin around cuticles.

4. **Cuticle stick** – to gently push back the cuticles.

5. **Base coat** – holds the color on the nail.

6. **Top coat** – seals the color in and protects the surface.

7. **Nail polish** – coloring as follows: cream for all occasions, high lacquer gloss for glamorous occasions, and frost for every occasion. Your nail color should match your lipstick – that is: blue nails do not go with red lipstick. Pick up your fashion cues from your garments.

8. **Cotton balls** – large balls for nail cleaning and polish removal.

The Basic Manicure – Ten Steps to Fabulous Nails

Step One. Start clean. Wash your hands. Wipe away all polish with an acetone-type polish remover.

Step Two. Shorten nails with a nail clipper before shaping. Shape your nails with a quality-grade emery board or file. Gently file the nail on both sides, moving in one direction toward the center.

Step Three. Soak fingers in a nail bowl, using warm soapy water, for several minutes and towel dry.

Step Four. Apply cuticle remover to the sides and base of nails and under nails. Gently push back cuticle with a manicure orange stick or cuticle shaper. Caution: Be extremely careful and focused when doing this procedure. You can cause discomfort and sensitivity around the cuticle if you push too hard. Furthermore, if you are too rough, you can create dark areas around the cuticle. Be gentle! Always sterilize the cuticle area with alcohol or peroxide to prevent swelling and infection. Remove excess cuticle remover lotion from your nails by soaking them in peroxide.

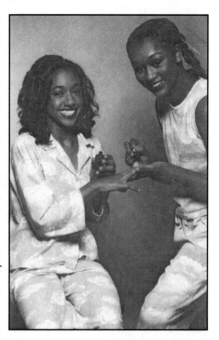

Step Five. Clipping excess cuticle and hangnails would be done if needed, but it is not usually recommended if you are not experienced. (If you must have it done, it's best left to a professional)

Step Six. Smooth the nail surface and edges with a quality buffer. If you feel the nail mantle (the surface0 getting warm and numb, you are removing too many layers of the nail. Be observant. If you take your time and concentrate, you can achieve nail salon perfection results. Remember to always buff in one direction.

Step Seven. Apply a clear base coat.

Step Eight. Apply two coats of nail polish: one broad stroke down the center and one on each side. Clean up any mess with a swab saturated in polish remover, or peroxide will do the trick.

Step Nine. Apply quick-drying or speed-drying spray to the nails.

Step Ten. Pamper your lovely nails with a hand-softening cream made with silky-smooth properties.

FYI

Got Hangnails?

If so, they are best left to a professional. But if you must treat them yourself, keep the nails clean and moist. Treat them to a little tea tree oil – great therapy!

Got Ridges and Stains?

Buffing can even out ridges on your nails and can aid in removing surface stains on your nails.

Different Special Effects for Your Nails

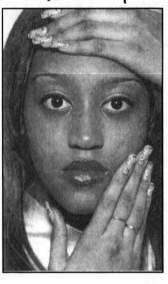

o Stencils come in a variety of cutout designs. After your nails are polished and dry, stick on your favorite shape, polish it and peel it off. Voila!

o Nail art is good if you or someone you know is an artist. Dream up any design you want and paint it on dry polished nails in contrasting colors.

o Decals are little design shapes that stick to or adhere to your nail. Apply them to clear or dry polished nails and then paint over them with a clear coat of polish or top coat.

o Jewels are little sparkly gems that you stick on for shimmery pizzazz. Apply them after you polish your nails and before they dry. Or to stick them on dry polish, use the special nail adhesive that comes in the kit.

o The French manicure is very chic and classy. To achieve this look, you first polish your nails in a neutral color like beige or light pink. Then you paint a coat of opaque white polish in a straight line across the tip of your nail. (Get help if you need it). If you can't draw straight, try a French manicure kit with stick-on stencils.

Beauty Notes

Weak, fragile, chipping, splitting and peeling nails require regular conditioning treatment, or liquid nail wrap is recommended. Always carry an emery board with you so you can get rid of snags right away. Keep your nails as short as you can stand until you treat them and make them stronger. The best way to do that is by massaging cuticle oil or a protein into them daily. Just use a clear protective polish until you see improvement.

Step Up With Glorious Feet

Gearing up for a pedicure? Here's what you need:
- Nail Polish Remover
- Cotton Balls or Pads
- Emery Board or Emery File
- Nail Soak
- Cuticle Lotion Remover
- Manicure Orange Stick
- Toenail clippers
- Pumice Stone or Foot Groomer
- Base Coat
- Nail Polish
- Quick-Drying or Speed-Drying Top Coat
- Creamy Foot-Moisturizing Conditioner

The Pedicure - Here's How:

To prepare for a pedicure, scrub your feet in the shower or bath, using a pumice stone or liquid rough-skin remover. This will gently smooth your feet.

- **Step One.** Remove old nail polish

- **Step Two.** Trim the toenails with toenail clippers. With an emery board or emery file, round the corners of the toenails.

o **Step Three to Ten.** (Follow the same steps given in the "Basic Manicure – Ten Steps to Fabulous Nails")

Special Stuff

o When you do housework (especially when using water) always wear rubber gloves.

o Artificial nails are in fashion and come in great colors. Yes, they can be fun. So, if you must, try them for special occasions.

o Your own nails will be strong and long if you manicure them every week.

o Make sure you eat a balanced diet. Calcium is good for your nails. Try milk, yogurt, cheese and broccoli.

o To soften your hands and feet, apply moisturizer and wear cotton socks or gloves to bed.

o Creams with natural ingredients, such as keratin, protein, and vitamin E are great for your hands and nails.

Ask Mercedes Fleetwood:

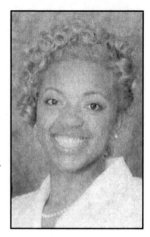

I am absolutely bored with my hair style! I want something that is low maintenance; and, most importantly, something that promotes hair health. What do you suggest?

Have you considered going natural? There are many ways to style your hair if it is chemical free. Start with a good cut, conditioner and moisturizing products. As your hair grows out, continue to clip the ends at least every six weeks. Eventually you will be able to train your hair to achieve the natural style you are most comfortable with.

Chapter Eight

Teen Talk Bonus Chapter: Special Things To Remember

Those Little Extras That Define You!

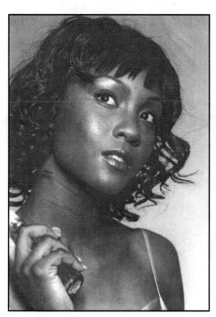

You're an individual. All the little things you do and wear make you stand out and help create your own special identity. You want to look good! Feel good! Smell good! You know everybody wants to! Here's how!

Smellin' Good – Making Sense of Your Fragrance Choices

It's about pleasing the senses. Fragrances can be silent, suggestive, and should reveal something about your personality and your moods.

Building Your Fragrance Collection

The average teenager owns or purchases four to eight different scents. These purchases are made from the oil perfume vendors on the street, department stores, chains, drugstores, mail order, and of course through the Internet.

No matter how you purchase it, you must take some time to select a scent. Some teenagers like to have a scent arrive before they do and the essence of that scent linger after the grand departure. Some boys like girls who really smell good. Certain fragrances evoke past, present, and future. Some of your girlfriends like the silent, understated, but suggestive scents with an edge. Do you know what scent brings out your beauty and allure.

Consider your body's chemistry. What smells great on your girlfriends and seems just right may not produce the same effect on you and others. Fragrance develops differently on individual skin types, depending on natural skin oils, body temperature, and the season. If your skin is oily and the weather is hot, and you have selected an intense perfume, it evaporates faster, so the scent smells much stronger. If your skin is dry and the fragrance is alcohol based, the fragrance sinks into the skin. You may have to reapply the fragrance several times to keep the scent potent.

Categories of Scent

o Floral is the power of one flower. Modern blends of flowers are called floral.

o Mossy green is reminiscent of a woodsy, outdoor autumn day, with combinations of ferns and herbs.

o Oriental scents are mysterious, sultry and exotic. They denote luxury and opulence. Some blends include musk, patchouli and sandalwood.

o   Spicy includes extracts of cinnamon, vanilla, ginger, carnation and cloves – the scent that tarries and hangs around.

o   Fruity fragrances are refreshing and light citrus blends. This happy mood scent includes bits of lemon, mandarin and lime.

Top note: First smell of the scent is called top note.

Middle Note: The main body of the fragrance. For example – woodsy, floral, Oriental and other.

Bottom note: The true essence of the scent, which lingers the longest, augmented by other aromatic blends.

Fragrance Classification

o   **Perfume** is the longest-lasting concentrated form of fragrance.

o   **Perfume Solid Formula** is one of the hottest concentrations that comes in a pot, solid cream, and a cream-to-powder compact.

o   **Perfume Oil** is another hot and popular concentration with teenagers. It's a real bargain when purchased from a street vendor who specializes in pure oil-based roll-on musk, for example.

o   **Eau de Parfum** is a less concentrated form of full-strength perfume.

o   **Eau de Toilette** is third in perfume intensity. It's excellent as an all over body splash or spray.

o   **Cologne** is the lightest and most subtle form of perfume, and has less strength than eau de toilette.

o   **Splash** and **Mist or Eau Fraiche** are the most refreshing and lightest forms of fragrances. They are excellent as an after shower or after bath all over body splash or mist. Most are alcohol free. They are great for school, sports and quick travel touch-ups.

How to Test a Fragrance

Apply a fragrance to the underside of your wrist. For dry skin types, wait five minutes, and for oily skin types, wait ten minutes to discern the middle note. Remember, it is not the initial sniff that you are evaluating.

After the other elements have evaporated, move away from the perfume area of the cosmetics counter. Now, take a good long sniff of the wrist with the applied fragrance; and if it smells good, make your choice. If there is the slightest tinge of bad odor, you should reconsider.

Fragrance in Your Life

After a stressing exam, part-time job, or sport or exercise workout, wouldn't it be nice to come into your room at home — or dorm, hotel, or night over your girlfriend's house — enlivened with your favorite fragrance? Fragrance helps to create a relaxing atmosphere.

Home and Dorm Room

For special occasions, try the real thing — a bunch of fragrant flowers! Set several potpourri-filled bowls by your bed, chest of drawers, bookshelves, computer desk, and windowsills for total fragrance meltdown… and buy scented drawer liners…for an extra special touch.

Fragrance in the Home

The following are suggested as great accents for your closet, bedroom and bath.

- o **Closet:** Scented sachets are still in!

- o **Home or dorm room**: Spray scents from a can on baseboards, in corners, around doorjambs and on throw rugs. Place sachet or scented soaps in your underwear drawer.

- o **Bath:** Keep scented soaps and potpourri in a basket, on display. Spray towel collections with the lightest fragrance formulas.

The Scented Bath

Start with soft music or environment mood sounds (try the sounds of a waterfall, ocean beach, or gentle stream), one or two scented candles, and a tall refreshing glass of your favorite flavored mineral water. Now, draw warm, tepid water (not hot), add bath oils or crystals, clear your mind, and then unwind and relax.

Here are some more soothing bath products to consider for future in-bath experiences:

- o **Dry-combination skin** – Bath Oils add moisturizing emollients and lubricants.

- o **Oily and troubled skin** – Bath gels are fine for those who miss soap. Gels clean the body gently and leave the body lightly scented and smooth.

- o **All skin types** – Herbal bath beads impart all-natural conditioning care. A milk bath softens and silkens the body. Bubble bath contains emollients to relax and soften the skin. Scented crystals are heavily scented, and most add harmless colors to the water.

Your Tools for Bathing

- o **Body Brush**

  Brings a nice healthy sheen to dark skin. Use a brush with natural bristles. Do not use rubber bath or synthetic bristles. (These bath tools will leave marks and cause uneven toned skin on most of us).

- o **Loufah**

  The loufah sloughs off dead skin cells, unclogs pores, softens and smoothes the skin. Our ancestors have used this body bathing tool for centuries. It is the dried seedpod of a tropical gourd.

- o **Other Bath Tools**

  The body cloth, friction mitt, and natural sea sponge are used for body cleansing and to help remove dead skin cells.

Quiz

LET'S NOW REVIEW and answer some of the most frequently asked questions about fragrances.

Q. Is fragrance enough?
A. Why not complement the many facets of your lifestyle? Spotlight these dimensions with special scents. Build a collection so you will have a fragrance for every occasion.

Q. Which perfume will be right for me?
A. Spray the fragrance on the underside of your wrist, wait about five to ten minutes, and then see how you like it. Make your choice.

Q. Where should I keep my perfume?
A. Keep your perfume away from heat and direct sunlight. Always keep the cap on to prevent evaporation.

Q. What is the difference between perfume, cologne and eau de toilette?
A. Perfume is the most potent of all, eau de toilette is second in perfume intensity, and cologne is the lightest, most subtle form of fragrance.

Q. Does body chemistry affect fragrance?
A. Whether you have oily, dry, or combination skin, the season of the year, the climate, and your body temperature all affect the performance of fragrance on your skin. Fragrances last longer on oily skin and in warm weather. In contrast, fragrance evaporates more rapidly on dry skin and in cold weather. No perfume smells exactly the same on two people.

Basic Beauty Facts
For strong, healthy nails, a high protein diet is best. It takes four to six months to grow a full-length new nail.

The 411 on Tattoos and Body Piercing

Tattooing: It's a Culture, Not Just a Trend

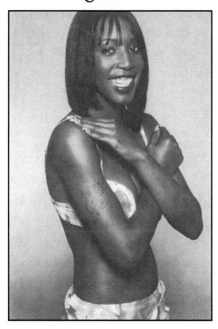

At one time, it was commonly thought that only people in motorcycle clubs and gangs wore tattoos. But rap, hip-hop, and R & B in our culture have opened up how a tattoo is viewed and valued by mainstream society. Social values are now more relaxed, and the tattoo has moved from being an "outsider" or "deviant" art form to being a more socially acceptable and admired art form. Tattoos have become more widely acceptable over the last ten years than in any other time in history. They have been popularized through their use in advertisements and by the BET and MTV crowd of the 1980s treading its way into the business offices of today's world. Tattoos can be seen as being status indicators, power symbols, worn by warriors, criminal brands, deviant icons, and even "fad" body accessories. Tattoos can also be used as symbols for a unique group, such as gangs, fraternities, or certain cultures. The tattoo has represented many things to many people in many places.

Tattooing can often be very beautiful and can be your personal statement about who you are. Tattooing can make you stand out in a crowd, giving you a special dimension of individuality, or it can be an indication of your culture. In fact, the art of tattooing has evolved in many cultures worldwide; and throughout history, it has been viewed in a variety of ways.

Henna has been used pretty expansively in the Middle East, where in places like Casablanca and Rabat, women – older women wearing djelibas, young women in smart suits, high school students in jeans – can be seen on the bus or walking through town wearing henna tattoos.

Henna and how and when it is used varies greatly from culture to culture. In Morocco, for instance, henna tattoos are quite prevalent, and the patterns vary distinctly. For instance, in rural areas, the designs are often cruder and thicker, with blunt designs and big geometric shapes, but in the cities, the designs are elaborate and very popular. Traditionally, a new bride, as well as all of her friends, has a big henna party where the bride gets most of the henna work and her friends get smaller designs on their hands and feet.

The art of tattooing has been transformed as a result of not only changes in social values but also those in power redefining mainstream values. Henna "tattoos" have traditionally been used by folkloric dancers, by Persian dancers, and by Native American tribal style troupes. Henna designs are so diverse that they can appear in whole-arm designs worn by certain cultures or groups, and they are worn on the upper arm by fashion models. Hennaed "bracelets" have become a great accessory; but if you use henna as a fashion statement, you have one prime consideration – henna is orange. If you think orange designs would go well with your fashions, go for it!

Temporary Tattoos to Consider.... Which Type of Henna is Best?

Stick with Natural or Traditional Henna. It is a natural plant dye that colors the skin orange/brown. It is safe because the dye in henna penetrates only as far as the outer dead skin cells – the epidermis. You can tell if your henna artist is using safe henna because the stain will be orange/brown and the paste will not be jet black. However, natural henna can go almost black in high heat and other safer ingredients exist. The artist should be able to tell you what ingredients have been used.

Black Henna Tattoos May be Hazardous to Your health. Teens who don't know the dangers connected with black henna sometimes prefer the black look as it looks similar to a permanent tattoo.

Black henna is a natural henna mixed with a black dye, which gives a long-lasting jet black color. This is because the dye used in black henna is PPD (phenylenediamine), a black chemical dye used as hair dye. Unfortunately, when applied to the skin it can cause an allergic reaction in some people – anything from a slight rash to blisters, oozing sores, intense itching, and long term scarring. Before you get any tattoo, always ask the artist what ingredients are being used. If they can't tell you, walk away. If they can, judge what they say for yourself. If the paste is jet black, walk away. If the stain is jet black, took less than two hours to go black and lasts for ten days or more, it's PPD.

Quick and Easy Tattoos:

You can make a statement with a temporary tattoo that is quick and easy to apply, and you can change the designs whenever you want a new look. (Check the ingredients to make sure there are no dye products that you are allergic to). Some of the designs you can get include: armbands, hearts and love, barbed wire, birds, butterflies, dragonflies, cartoon characters, crosses, stars, moons, dragons, snakes, superheroes, flowers, tribal designs and wild beasts. For teenagers, this is probably the best way to go.

Consider This!

Body tattooing can be very painful, and it is permanent. Lasers can remove them, although quite often, it just lightens the tattoo. They can be surgically removed, but then you are left with a scar and if your skin has a tendency to keloid, that could be disastrous. It's definitely not safe to tattoo the breast of nipple area, and to consider tattooing the vaginal area is horrific. If you are under the age of eighteen, definitely do not run off and get a permanent tattoo – your parents would probably never forgive you!

Body Piercing

Just like tattooing, body piercing has cultural roots. Body modification, enhancement, and adornment have all been a part of human culture throughout history. It's an art form that has been used by hundreds of tribes throughout the world for centuries, often used as a status symbol. Naval piercing was a symbol of royalty among ancient Egyptians. Amazonian tribal hunters and gatherers wore bull rings to look more fearsome so they could intimidate their prey. A lot of girls get body piercings because their friends do. Again, consider your uniqueness, when choosing this accessory, and use good judgment to decide when and where to pierce.

Food and Fitness for a Better You

Many facets are involved in making you as beautiful as you are. We've talked extensively about your skin, makeup, and hair. Let's spend a little time now on your physical self – being fit and fabulous!

Fast Break

The most important meal – hands down – is BREAKFAST! After resting (or fasting) all night, your body now needs to be refueled and reenergized to meet the needs of a new day. Don't make a "fast break" for the door without stopping for refueling; take time to "break the fast."

A Few Quick Healthy Choices
- Bowl of hot or cold cereal with milk (try soy milk, you might like it), topped with fruit.
- Bagel with melted cheese or peanut butter, and fruit or juice.
- Yogurt parfait (alternate layers of plain/lemon/vanilla yogurt) with fruit and topped with cereal (such as granola).

Snacks

Snacks can be a quick-and-easy way to refuel your body. Just remember that frequent snacking also means you are increasing your caloric intake. Snacks should not replace meals.

Quick Pick-Me-Up-Snacks

o   Cottage cheese/fruit

o   Yogurt parfait

o   Flavored rice cakes or corn cakes, with peanut butter.

o   Apple slices and cheese slices.

o   Homemade trail mix. Add or delete the foods of your choice:
    ¼ cup low-sugar cereal (add Kix or Cheerios)
    ¼ cup nuts/seeds (add sunflower seeds, peanuts or almonds)
    ¼ cup dried fruit and raisins? Maybe!
    ¼ cup pretzels

Got a Sweet Tooth?

o   Desserts are a wonderful part of your diet, and you need not deny yourself. Just don't overdo them. When you have the great sweet urge, consider one of the following.

o   Sweet Treats

o   Angel food cake with fresh strawberries

o   Small bowl of ice cream topped with fresh fruit

o   Muffins, banana bread, cranberry bread, zucchini bread

o   Fruit salad

o   Half a grapefruit with a sprinkling of sugar

o   *Homemade* milkshake with fruit (combine skim milk with ice milk or low fat ice cream).

Watch Out for Weight Gain

o Limit sweets and fatty foods

o Choose snacks wisely. Avoid mountains of empty-calorie foods such as chips, cookies, candy bars. They are full of calories but low in nutrients. The closer a food is to its natural state, the healthier it usually is for you.

o If your favorite food is also high in fat, don't deny yourself; just don't eat it daily.

o Read nutrition labels carefully. The higher the number of in-gredients, the more processed (refined) it may be. This removes many vitamins that may not be added back. The less processed the food, the lower it is in fat.

o Watch out for "sneaky calories." These are sneaky because they taste good and are high in calories, but provide little or no nutrition. For that reason, salad dressing, mayonnaise, butter, sugar and oils should all be used sparingly.

o Beware of "liquid calories." Drinks like soda pop and café lattes, are full of sneaky calories. Reading labels is a *must!* If a label uses punch, cocktail or –ade, then sugar has been added.

How Your Body Uses Water

o Mode of transportation for nutrients to enter the cells.
o Mode of transportation for waste products to exit the body.
o Shock absorber, joint lubricant, and much more!

Is it hard to imagine drinking six to eight glasses a day? Try bottled fla-vored waters. These are cheaper per bottle than soda pop when bought by the case. Or add a slice of lemon or lime to your water. Or make your own flavored water by mixing carbonated water with a little 100 percent fruit juice. Fluids from other drinks such as juice and tea do count. Just remember to choose caffeine-free drinks, because caffeine does act as a diuretic in the body, flushing the needed water right out, thus increasing your need for water even more.

Try Vegetarian Nutrician

Vegetarians do not eat meat, fish or poultry. Most vegetarians abstain from eating or using all animal products, including milk, cheese, other dairy items, and eggs. Among the many reasons for being a vegetarian are your health, ecological and religious concerns, dislike for meat, compassion for animals, belief in nonviolence, and economics.

The key to a healthy vegetarian diet, as with any other diet, is to eat a wide variety of foods, including fruits, vegetables, plenty of leafy greens, whole grain products, nuts, seeds and legumes.

For a Healthy Vegetarian Diet, Variety is the Key

The most important concern for teenage vegetarians is the nutritional adequacy of their food choices. A vegetarian diet can be enjoyed by people of all ages, but the key to a healthy vegetarian diet is variety. Just as your parents would be concerned if you ate only hamburgers, they would also worry if you eat only potato chips and salad. A healthy and varied vegetarian diet includes fruits, vegetables, plenty of leafy greens, whole grain products, nuts, seeds and legumes. Some vegetarians also choose to eat dairy products and/or eggs.

Teenage vegetarians have nutritional needs that are the same as any other teenager. The years between thirteen and nineteen are times of especially rapid growth and change, so additional needs are high during these years. The nutrients that you will probably be asked about the most are protein, calcium, iron and vitamin B12.

What About Protein?

Cow's milk and low-fat cheese are protein sources; however, beans, breads, cereals, nuts, peanut butter, tofu, and soy milk are also some foods that are especially good sources of protein. Fruits, fats and sugars do not provide much protein, so a diet based only on these foods would probably be too low in protein. It is not necessary to plan combinations of foods to obtain enough protein or amino acids, which are components of protein. A mixture of plant proteins eaten throughout the day will provide enough amino acids.

Other Important Nutrients

Especially during adolescence, calcium is needed to build bones. Bone density is determined in adolescence and young adulthood, so it is important to include three or more good sources of calcium in your diet every day. Cow's milk and dairy products do contain calcium. However, there are other good sources of calcium sulfate: tahini (sesame butter); green leafy vegetables, including collard greens, mustard greens, and kale; calcium-fortified soy milk and orange juice.

Iron requirements of teenagers are relatively high. By eating a vegetarian diet, a vegetarian can meet iron needs while avoiding the excess fat and cholesterol found in red meats, such as beef or pork. To increase the amount of iron absorbed from meat, eat a food containing vitamin C as part of the meal. Citrus fruits and juices (for example, orange juice), tomatoes, and broccoli are all good sources of vitamin C. Foods that are high in iron include broccoli, raisins, watermelon, spinach, black-eyed peas, blackstrap molasses, chickpeas and pinto beans. Vegetarians need to add vitamin B12 to their diet. Some cereals, such as Grape-Nuts, and fortified soymilks have vitamin B12, (check the label).

Getting Fit With Your Favorite Exercises

Look at your body and decide which areas need the most work. In addition to reducing the body's fat reserves and building energy, exercise keeps you fit, relaxes you, and helps you to manage stress better. The key ingredients for establishing a successful exercise regimen are discipline and consistency. Begin by finding a convenient place where you can work out. Try to do at least fifteen to twenty minutes of exercise before you start your day. If you have time before or after school, you could workout on your bedroom floor, on your patio or in your yard. Make sure you'll have the tools you'll need, such as hand weights, a fitness mat, and maybe a jump-rope or step bench. If you have a break during the day, perhaps you can go to a nearby park, a health club, or a gym. You might be able to do a set of abdominal curls, push-ups, or arm exercises using weights. Whatever form of exercise you choose, remember, you can make it a habit if you always keep it convenient and practical.

Beauty Note
Body stretch marks around the neck, armpits, stomach, buttocks, and thigh areas, which may appear after weight loss, body shaping or body building are often hereditary. If they begin to appear, apply cocoa butter on the areas several times a day, (whenever possible), which often lessens the extent of the discoloration.

All in the Game of Sports

For active teens, diet and nutrition are very important. Many of you are playing competitive high school sports and may be preparing to carry this skill into the college women's tournaments in competition. If you are an athlete, you are likely to perspire excessively, and therefore you should shower and shampoo a lot.

Moisturizing dehydrated skin is very important for your overall appearance, as well as conditioning your hair daily. The following regimen is recommended:

- o Cleanse
- o Tone
- o Moisturize
- o Apply no foundation
- o Use a little waterproof smear-proof mascara
- o Use lip-liner pencil to match a sheer lipstick color

If you are physically active, eat a great diet and follow this regular skincare routine, you'll look and feel fabulous.

Rest and Relaxation

One of the most important things you can do as a teenager is to value sleep. If you feel tired and there is an opportunity to nap during the day, take it. This doesn't mean you should fall asleep in history class, but that you should take a quick snooze after school, before practice. Your naps shouldn't last any longer than an hour and should be planned ahead of time. Falling asleep while trying to do your homework is not a scheduled nap. But, if you decide to come home from school, eat a snack, and sleep for forty-five minutes; that will help you control your tiredness.

If you're an athlete who has an important competition coming up in a few days, try to get nine hours of sleep on the nights leading up to the event. If nerves keep you up the night before, at least you'll have a few good nights of sleep in the bank. On the night of your game, try to get your homework done in between classes and before the event. That way, instead of coming home exhausted after the game and trying to get your homework done, you'll be able to go straight to bed, which will allow you to get a few more hours of sleep.

In order to get to bed at a reasonable time and fall asleep right away, stay away from the Internet or television before going to bed. Those pre-bedtime rituals may keep your energy up instead of letting your body wind down. Read instead.

Once the alarm goes off, get up and get moving – especially outside – ASAP. This is a great time to take a walk or do some stretches. Getting into the light right away will help reset your biological clock and let your body know it's time to wake up.

Sleep patterns are developed early in life, so your teen years are a great time to set standards that your body will follow for the rest of your life.

Massage

Massage can be a wonderful therapy. It helps you to relax your muscles, improves circulation, and cleanses the body of toxins. The best time to give yourself a massage is right after you bathe.

Start with your feet, the part of your body that works the hardest. They carry you around all day, and you seldom treat them well. After you bathe, spend a little time applying moisturizing cream to your legs, ankles, and toes. Work the lotion in well between your toes and up and down your legs.

Your arms are next. Apply lotion and firmly work it up and down your arms and shoulders. Continue to massage or knead your arms until you feel all the tension released, then work your way up to your shoulders.

Also massage the other fleshy areas of your body, such as your abdomen and thighs.

….or, better yet, whenever possible…go out to a spa and treat yourself to a professional massage. ***ENJOY!***

Take Good Care of Yourself
Every day, pause and take time to relax spiritually, physically, and mentally. Spend quiet time relaxing and tension that you might have. Breathe silently and deeply and meditate with your eyes shut.

Ask Mercedes Fleetwood:

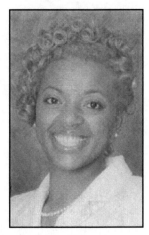

How do I pick a fragrance that smells great on me?

Complete your presentation with your favorite fragrance. It should compliment your mood and captivate those that you encounter. Avoid too strong scents that overpower you – it should be just enough to be pleasing and have a slightly lingering effect. When you find a fragrance that does all that, spray or dab it on your wrists, the curve of your neck and behind your ears – the pulse points are perfect. Stick to one fragrance at a time – never mix your scents.

Beauty Questions? Ask Mercedes Fleetwood ...email amberbk@aol.com

In Conclusion...

Be Proud of Yourself—You were Born Beautiful!

Always remember that good looks must be accompanied by facial expressions that reveal warmth and sincere friendliness. Attractive facial expressions add a glow that can make you stand out in a crowd. A lively smile and sparkling eyes will attract attention, and a face that mirrors a warm and kindly personality has a vivacious quality far more desirable than mere beauty.

Let your eyes show joy when you are happy about something and they will delight others as well. Maintain a warm and pleasing voice, whenever possible. Know your grammar, and expose yourself to good speech. Work on your pitch, enunciation, and pronunciation.

Just as water keeps your body strong, replenishing it with needed nutrients, so does fresh air keep your lungs strong and help them to breathe more clearly. Good breathing habits make a world of difference in both health and speech. Sit straight and stand tall at all times.

Finally, be proud of yourself! You were Born Beautiful! No matter what your age — from the young teen to the senior matron — all of you are *Ageless Beauties*.

God bless you!

Yvonne Rose

Ageless Beauty

About the Authors

Alfred Fornay

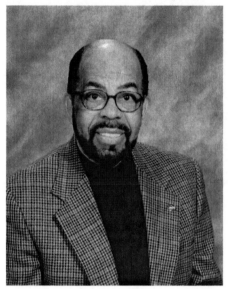

Alfred Fornay is one of the leading recognized authorities on fashion, beauty and grooming. A graduate of the State University of New York's Fashion Institute of Technology and the University of New York, with degrees in merchandising and marketing, Mr. Fornay has influenced the marketing and sales strategies of several major cosmetic firms, such as Fashion Fair, Clairol and Revlon. He was the Assistant Ethnic Marketing Manager for Clairol Cosmetics, Beauty/Training Director for Fashion Fair and Creative Director for Revlon's "Polished Ambers" Collection. Fornay is the guru of make up and skin care for a generation of women of color throughout the world.

Yvonne Rose

Yvonne Rose is the Associate Publisher and Senior Editor at Amber Communications Group, Inc., the nation's largest African-American publisher of Self-Help Books and Music Biographies. Ms. Rose began her stint at Amber Books as the co-author of the Company's flagship title, the national bestseller, *Is Modeling for You? The Handbook and Guide for the Young Aspiring Black Model.*

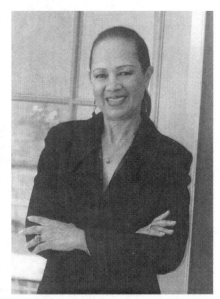

Founded in 1998 by Tony Rose, Publisher/CEO, Amber Communications Group, Inc., ACGI's imprints include: the award winning Amber Books Publishing — Self Help Books; Colossus Books — Music Biographies; Amber/Wiley Books — Self Help and Financial Books Co-Published with John Wiley & Sons Inc.; Joyner/Amber Books — Co-Published with the Tom Joyner Foundation and Legacy Books — Historic True Stories by African American Senior Citizens.

In January 2000 Tony Rose established Quality Press, a special service division for authors who wanted to self-publish their books instead of waiting to gain an interest from mainstream publishers. Yvonne was appointed Director of Quality Press and has turned hundreds of manuscripts into completed books.

Prior to entering the book publishing industry, Yvonne was an award-winning journalist who worked as a national model, and publicist, fashion and beauty editor for several national magazines. Yvonne has ghost-written and co-written numerous top selling non-fiction titles.

Order Form

Fax Orders:	480-283-0991
Telephone Orders:	602-743-7211
Online orders:	WWW.AMBERBOOKS.COM
Email:	Amberbk@aol.com

Postal Mail Orders: Send Checks & Money Orders
Payable to Amber Books
c/o Amber Communications Group, Inc
1334 East Chandler Boulevard, Suite 5-D67
Phoenix, AZ 85048

Please send _____ copy/ies of *Ageless Beauty: The Ultimage Skin Care & Makeup Book for Women & Teens of Color* by Alfred Fornay and Yvonne Rose - $15.95

Please send _____ copy/ies of *Is Modeling for You? The Handbook and Guide for the Young Aspiring Black Model* by Yvonne Rose and Tony Rose - $15.95

Please send _____ copy/ies of *Beautiful Black Hair: Real Solutions to Real* Problems by Shamboosie - $16.95

Please send _____ copy/ies of *The Afrocentric Bride: A Styling Guide* by Therez Fleetwood - $16.95

Please send _____ copy/ies of *Born Beautiful: The African American Teenagers Complete Beauty Guide* by Alfred Fornay - $14.95

Please send _____ copy/ies of *The African American Women's Guide to Successful Makeup & Skin Care* by Alfred Fornay - $16.95

Name: _____

Address: _____

City: _____ State: _____ Zip: _____

Phone: (_____)_____ Email: _____

Add $5 shipping per book
Sales tax: Add 7.05% to books shipped to Arizona addresses.

Total enclosed: $_____

Paid by:
- ❏ Check/Money order
- ❏ Credit Card #:_____ exp: _____

For Bulk Rates, Call: (602) 743-7211 or email: amberbk@aol.com

CPSIA information can be obtained at www.ICGtesting.com
Printed in the USA
LVOW131736020812

292692LV00015B/54/P